D1765220

Textbook of
PERIMENOPAUSAL
GYNECOLOGY

Textbook of
PERIMENOPAUSAL
GYNECOLOGY

Edited by

NANETTE SANTORO, MD   and   **STEVEN R. GOLDSTEIN**, MD
Albert Einstein College of Medicine   New York University School of Medicine,
of Yeshiva University, New York, NY, USA   New York, NY, USA

The Parthenon Publishing Group
International Publishers in Medicine, Science & Technology

A CRC PRESS COMPANY
BOCA RATON   LONDON   NEW YORK   WASHINGTON, D.C.

Dedication

This book is dedicated to Luke Goldstein whose actions continually remind me just how much a person can accomplish if they possess perseverance.

Library of Congress Cataloging-in-Publication Data

Data available on request

British Library Cataloguing in Publication Data
Textbook of perimenopausal gynecology
1. Gynecology 2. Perimenopause
I. Santoro, Nanette II. Goldstein, Steven R.
618.1

ISBN 1-84214-170-8

Published in the USA by
The Parthenon Publishing Group
345 Park Avenue South
10th Floor
New York, NY 10010, USA

Published in the UK and Europe by
The Parthenon Publishing Group
23–25 Blades Court
Deodar Road
London SW15 2NU, UK

Copyright © 2003
The Parthenon Publishing Group

No part of this book may be reproduced in any form without permission from the publishers, except for the quotation of brief passages for the purposes of review.

Typeset by Siva Math Setters, Chennai, India
Printed and bound by Bookcraft (Bath) Ltd.,
Midsomer Norton, UK

Contents

List of contributors   vii

Preface   ix

Foreword   xi

I.   Physiology of the menopause

1   Is it perimenopause? Diagnostic considerations   1
    N. Santoro

2   Reproductive aging: compensated ovarian failure   5
    N. A. Klein and M. R. Soules

3   Hormonal patterns in the later menopause transition   13
    H. Burger and N. Santoro

4   Body composition changes in midlife   19
    C. K. Sites

5   Studying the complexity of the menopause transition
    from an epidemiological perspective   27
    M. F. Sowers

6   Midlife sexuality   37
    A. Altman

II.   Signs and symptoms of perimenopause

7   Symptoms of the perimenopause   59
    L. Dennerstein and J. Guthrie

8   Bleeding patterns in perimenopausal women   69
    S. R. Goldstein

9   Screening for major malignancies in the perimenopausal woman   79
    V. A. Givens and F. W. Ling

10   Uterine disease in midlife women   87
    R. L. Barbieri

III.   Therapeutic considerations in the perimenopause

11   Creative use of oral contraceptives in the perimenopausal patient   99
    P. J. Sulak

12   Reduction of breast cancer risk in midlife women   109
    S. R. Goldstein

13 Minimal access surgery for uterine disease   119
    R. S. Neuwirth

14 Perimenopause: nutritional considerations   127
    J. Lovejoy and M. Hamilton

15 Hormonal management of symptoms   145
    J. L. Chervenak

Index   159

List of contributors

A. Altman
Department of Obstetrics, Gynecology and
  Reproductive Biology
Harvard Medical School
Boston
Massachusetts
USA

R. L. Barbieri
Department of Obstetrics and Gynecology
ASBI-3, Brigham and Women's Hospital
75 Francis Street
Boston, MA 02115
USA

H. Burger
Prince Henry's Institute of Medical
  Research
PO Box 5152
Clayton, Victoria 3168
Australia

J. L. Chervenak
Division of Reproductive Endocrinology
Albert Einstein College of Medicine
1300 Morris Park Avenue
Bronx, NY 10461
USA

L. Dennerstein
Office for Gender and Health
Department of Psychiatry
University of Melbourne
Royal Melbourne Hospital
Charles Connibere Building
Parkville, Victoria 3050
Australia

V. A. Givens
Department of Obstetrics and Gynecology
Division of Gynecologic Specialties
University of Tennessee Health
  Science Center
Room E-102, 853 Jefferson Avenue
Memphis, TN 38163
USA

S. R. Goldstein
Department of Obstetrics and Gynecology
New York University Medical Center
Suite 10N, 530 First Avenue
New York, NY 10016
USA

J. Guthrie
Office for Gender and Health
Department of Psychiatry
University of Melbourne
Royal Melbourne Hospital
Charles Connibere Building
Parkville, Victoria 3050
Australia

M. Hamilton
Pennington Biomedical Research Center
6400 Perkins Road
Baton Rouge, LA 70808
USA

N. A. Klein
Division of Reproductive Endocrinology
University of Washington
Suite 305, 4225 Roosevelt Way NE
Seattle, WA 98105
USA

F. W. Ling
Department of Obstetrics and
  Gynecology
University of Tennessee
Room E-102, 853 Jefferson Ave,
Memphis, TN 38103
USA

J. Lovejoy
Pennington Biomedical Research Center
6400 Perkins Road
Baton Rouge, LA 70808
USA

R. S. Neuwirth
St. Luke's–Roosevelt Hospital Center
Roosevelt Hospital
Suite 5A, 425 West 59th Street
New York, NY 10019
USA

N. Santoro
Division of Reproductive Endocrinology
Department of Obstetrics, Gynecology and
  Women's Health
Albert Einstein College of Medicine
1300 Morris Park Avenue
Bronx, NY 10461
USA

C. K. Sites
University of Vermont College of Medicine
Department of Obstetrics and Gynecology
Given Building C252
Burlington, VT 05405
USA

M. R. Soules
Division of Reproductive Endocrinology
University of Washington
Suite 305, 4225 Roosevelt Way NE
Seattle, WA 98105
USA

M. F. Sowers
School of Public Health
University of Michigan
109 Observatory Street
Ann Arbor, MI 48109
USA

P. J. Sulak
Texas A&M University Health Science Center
Department of Obstetrics and Gynecology
Scott & White Clinic/Memorial Hospital
2401 S. 31st Street
Temple, TX 76508
USA

Preface

Our patients are confused. Many physicians are confused. Labels like perimenopause, menopause and postmenopause are applied to a variety of clinical situations. This book was produced to help fill in some serious gaps in the knowledge base and practice of gynecology. It is tightly focused on women who are of reproductive age yet still premenopausal, a forgotten group of women who have varying health needs. Some are trying to conceive, and request advice about how best to maximize the twilight years of their fertility. Others are equally enthusiastically trying *not* to conceive, and request reassurance about the best ways to manage their contraceptive issues in the face of declining fertility and, perhaps, intermittent sexual relationships.

In many areas of health, women in this 'midlife zone' represent a challenging mixture of symptoms, hormones, preclinical and even clinical diseases. A practitioner who cares for such women needs to be prepared for tremendous variability. The clinician needs to be able to help a woman separate 'change' from disease, and needs to understand when symptoms or problems are likely to be due to the menopausal transition and when they are likely to be due to aging or unhealthy long-term lifestyle habits. This book is designed to help clinicians make these distinctions.

We present this material to you in three major sections. Section I covers the exciting field of research into the perimenopause, or the menopause transition. A series of reproductive hormonal events precedes the development of follicle failure and anovulation, and recent scientific evidence on populations of women is turning up important information critical to the understanding of clinical management. Our authors are all primary researchers in these areas. We think you will find what they have to say to be very illuminating. This was not presented previously in your studies or training simply because it was not known. In the second section, some key, common symptomatology is discussed. From a gynecological point of view, bleeding issues tend to dominate the discussion, but it is important to note that, as gynecologists, we have the opportunity to intervene in many more areas of symptomatology and to help our patients clarify which symptoms may be amenable to hormonal interventions. Finally, some guidelines for management of bothersome symptoms and frequently asked questions and concerns of women in their middle years are discussed. Please keep in mind that therapeutics in this area are a work in progress. New developments are happening almost daily.

A book like this does not happen without the dedicated work of its authors, each one of whom was asked to provide the most up-to-date material. This made the work of the Editors easy, and we are proud to present this manual to you.

Steven R. Goldstein, MD
New York, NY

Nanette Santoro, MD
New York, NY

Foreword

Barely 40 years ago the subject of menopause was no more than a one-liner in a general textbook of gynecology, reading, 'menopause is physiological amenorrhea'. The last four decades have witnessed huge strides in relation to our understanding of the menopause transition and the years beyond the menopause. Above all, the basic physiopathology is being elucidated, the changing demographics and its impact on the healthcare industry better understood, and yet many questions remain.

Appropriate use of language is extremely important, and this is a book on the perimenopause. The Council of Affiliated Menopause Societies defined perimenopause as 'the time immediately prior to the menopause (when the endocrinological, biological, and clinical features of approaching menopause commence) and the first year after menopause'. In this volume, Drs Goldstein and Santoro have co-ordinated contributions from an extremely distinguished group of medical scientists, investigators and clinicians. The definition of perimenopause is then fully 'fleshed out' into the physiological, clinical and therapeutic considerations.

The question of whether the perimenopause requires some form of pharmacotherapy remains debatable, essentially as the issues regarding hormone replacement therapy become ever more controversial. Unfortunately, the largest of the recent randomized prospective studies, notably that of the Women's Health Initiative and the HERS study, have not addressed the population in the perimenopause, and do not clarify the role of hormone therapies. Nor is it yet clear what the role of other preventive modalities should be.

Fortunately, the background to the above debate is well described within the body of this book and it will, therefore, be of significant value not only to practitioners involved in the care of women through and beyond menopause, but, indeed, should be part of required reading for residents-in-training, and a broad array of medical specialties.

The perimenopause represents a clinical challenge to the modern practitioner in that it offers opportunities for identification of early risk factors of future disease, indicators of early presence of established disease, and an opportunity to enhance the quality of care for women in their later years.

Wulf H. Utian, MD, PhD
Executive Director, The North American Menopause Society
Consultant Gynecologist, The Cleveland Clinic
President, Rapid Medical Research Inc.

Acknowledgements

No matter how many books I have written the process of sitting down and collecting my thoughts about how a volume came to be, and then being able to acknowledge those involved is still a most gratifying experience. Those people include Nat Russo at Parthenon Publishing, an old friend and a new motivator; Nanette Santoro, as bright and honest a co-writer as one could ever hope for, and my first and only choice during this volume's gestational period; Laurie Ashner, my co-writer in my lay book on perimenopause, whose constant questions always cause me to see things in a slightly different light; Gary Mucciolo MD and my staff, Christine Sweeney, Mercy Faraci, Juanita Castro and Beverly Shamah, whose wonderful organization of my clinical coverage has enabled me to accomplish what I have; Penny Franco, my academic right hand who keeps me on the straight and narrow; my patients, those wonderful patients, whose demanding but articulate nature enabled me to understand so much about perimenopause; my children, Phoebe Jordan and Austin Lucas (Luke) who daily make me realize they are the reason we keep going; but most of all my wife, Kathy Dillon Goldstein who continues to be my life partner and enables me to do what I do and be who I am.

Steven R. Goldstein, MD

As this is the first book for which I've been responsible, I must thank Nat Russo from Parthenon Publishing for getting Steve and myself together and helping us make a series of topically important chapters take shape. Next, of course, comes Steve Goldstein, who was a joy to work with. Our chapter authors provided us with the best possible material for the book (which is why we chose them), and to them all I owe great gratitude. My secretary, Edith Rodriguez, deserves credit for her work in tracking the progress, and sometimes the authors. Finally, to my family, Alan, Amanda and Russell, who put up with my deadlines and endless lists of projects, I give my love and dedication.

Nanette Santoro, MD

Is it perimenopause? Diagnostic considerations

1

N. Santoro

Current demographics of the menopause

The median age at menopause has been stable in recorded studies over the past 100 years. This is in contrast to the median age at menarche, which has demonstrated a continuing decline since it began to be systematically measured[1]. Based on recent studies of women in the USA, the onset of cycle irregularity associated with the menopause transition begins at around age 47 and lasts for 2–4 years[2,3]. There is considerable variation about this median, with a skewing towards earlier ages. It is not unusual for a woman to have her final menstrual period prior to the age of 45; about 5% of women experience menopause this early[4,5]. It also appears that the earlier the cycle irregularity begins, the longer the duration of the transition. Therefore, a woman who begins to have irregular cycles at age 38–40 may continue to cycle intermittently until she is well into her late forties. Stated another way, an early onset of the menopause transition does not necessarily predict an early final menstrual period.

There are several non-reproductive factors known to influence the timing and perhaps the tempo of the menopausal transition. Cigarette smoking advances the age at menopause by approximately 2–4 years and is the largest single environmental factor that has been identified[3,6]. It is controversial whether or not smoking cessation in older reproductive-aged women reduces or eliminates this effect; the most recent population-based data from a US study have indicated that the effect can be appreciably modified by smoking cessation at any stage[3]. Psychosocial stress and low socioeconomic status predict earlier menopause[7,8]. A history of medically treated depression appears also to be linked to earlier menopause[9]. Family history is also a predictor of early menopause in women[10].

The likelihood that a woman is menopausal is based in part upon her age and in part upon the duration of amenorrhea[11]. In a review of the Treloar database, Wallace and co-workers established some limits that are helpful in defining the transition. Women over the age of 45 who have been amenorrheic for at least 12 months have a 90% probability of never having another menstrual period. This constitutes the current clinical working definition of menopause, and it is arrived at retrospectively. This definition also indicates that 12 months of amenorrhea is not an absolute criterion; menses may still occur after this apparent milestone has been achieved, in one of ten women. Importantly, age appears to exert a mitigating influence on the probability of menopause. Women with prolonged amenorrhea who are younger than 45 years are not part of this definition and may have a much greater likelihood of regaining some menstrual cyclicity in the future. This information is useful when counselling patients about the likelihood of future cycling.

Prospective studies of women traversing the menopause have yielded some epidemiologically validated 'stages'. A woman is considered to have entered the menopause transition when she either notes increased irregularity and unpredictability of her cycles or starts to 'skip' cycles[12,13]. The 'early' menopause transition is defined as less than 3 months of consecutive amenorrhea in a woman who had been cycling regularly in her mid-reproductive years. The 'early' menopause transition appears to be the most variable in length. The 'late' menopause transition is defined as 3–11 months of amenorrhea. Garamszegi and associates analyzed data on hundreds of women in a prospective cohort of women in Melbourne, Australia. Using prospectively collected menstrual calendars, similar to that of Treloar, they were able to demonstrate that bouts of prolonged amenorrhea (defined as at least three but not more than 11 consecutive months) predicted that the final menstrual period would occur in 95% of women within the following 4 years[14]. While these definitions are relatively crude and lack the precision that clinicians might like to be able to give their patients, they are currently the best available.

The final menstrual period is defined when 12 consecutive months of amenorrhea have been attained. There is virtually no information that can guide the clinician when counselling women who do not have regular menstrual cycles. Interestingly, in some of these conditions, such as polycystic ovary syndrome, the hormonal changes that accompany the transition may favor more regular cyclicity in women in their mid- to late forties.

Clinical signs and symptoms of the perimenopause

Several worldwide studies of perimenopausal symptomatology have provided somewhat similar data. Symptoms of the menopause transition appear to be broad, vague and generally non-specific. It is not clear that a symptom complex easily attributable to the menopause transition exists. Moreover, there are large differences in symptom reporting between clinic-based and population-based cohorts. Data from the Massachusetts Women's

Health Study suggested that approximately 50% of women sought medical consultation for their menopausal symptoms and that most of these women sought consultation before their final menstrual period[2]. An analysis of perimenopausal symptoms carried out longitudinally has been recently reported by Dennerstein and colleagues. The most significant changes in symptoms that occurred as women traversed the menopause were that symptoms of breast tenderness and headache decreased while symptoms of hot flashes, night sweats and genitourinary atrophy increased[15].

The eloquence and precision with which some patients are able to attribute specific symptoms to changes in their menstrual cycles is not supported by grouped data from many women. Prospective symptom studies may need to be better designed to identify subgroups of women prone to specific complexes of symptoms. There is evidence that the perimenopausal years engender some loss of quality of life for many women. Some may simply feel a 'loss of wellness'. There is evidence that homeostasis is attained during or after the transition, but there may be temporary adversity associated with some symptoms. On the other hand, an appreciable number of women traverse the menopause without any symptoms.

Contrary to popular belief, the prevalence of depression was not shown to rise at any point during the transition in population-based studies[2]. However, women with a history of depression may be more vulnerable to recurrence of symptoms and may present to the clinician at this time[9]. Women who are depressed may also be disproportionately represented in physicians' offices[16]. It is difficult but important to maintain the perspective that the prevalence of patients' complaints within an office practice is not the same as the population prevalence.

Because many of the symptoms reported by perimenopausal women are non-specific, attention should be paid to other potential medical conditions that could cause the same symptomatology. Depression is a common confounder for listlessness and fatigue, and thyroid screening should be considered to rule out hypothyroidism. Sleep complaints are often, but not uniformly, attributable to hot flashes/night sweats. Sleep quality declines with age and, especially in obese women, sleep apnea should be considered. This is especially true if hormone therapy does not have a salutary impact on poor sleep. Many rare entities that can present in the perimenopausal period and are therefore worth considering include primary adrenal failure, Cushing's disease, fibromyalgia, chronic fatigue syndrome and possibly secondary Lyme disease, when the presenting problems center on fatigue. Women with hot flashes who do not respond to hormonal treatment may be suffering from panic disorder, diabetic autonomic dysfunction, hyperventilation, or even pheochromocytoma or carcinoid syndrome.

How is the diagnosis made?

A reasonable diagnostic paradigm for a perimenopausal woman with adverse symptomatology starts with an assessment of her age and menstrual pattern. If she is 45 years or older, has increased irregularity of her menses or skipped cycles, and at least some symptoms suggestive of hypoestrogenism (mild hot flashes or night sweats), then a presumptive diagnosis of perimenopause is possible without further evaluation. Patients with symptoms of fatigue should be investigated further with a screen for depression and a screening thyroid stimulating hormone level, if one has not been performed recently. Women under the age of 40 with perimenopausal symptoms and amenorrhea for longer than 3 months are likely to have premature ovarian failure. These women should be screened further with antithyroid and antiadrenal antibodies, routine chemistries and hematologies to rule out some of the autoimmune disorders associated with premature menopause[17]. Other autoimmune

screening or karyotyping can be performed as indicated. Women between these age groups may simply be presenting with early menopause, but other possible diagnoses should be considered. Only 5% of the population experience menopause prior to age 45[4].

A small percentage of women are chronically hypogonadotropic and oligomenorrheic, and detection of the menopausal transition in these women can be challenging. For example, women who abuse alcohol or street drugs have been shown to have elevated prolactin and relative hypogonadotropism[18]. The effects that these processes have on the menopause transition is not known, but the elevated prolactin does appear to be associated with decreased FSH[19].

Summary

The menopause transition appears to be a stressor for many, if not most, women. The spectrum of symptoms and their severity vary greatly from woman to woman. To make matters more confusing, the menopausal process, as well as its symptoms, may pursue a waxing and waning course. Congruent signs and symptoms favor the simple diagnosis of perimenopause, and many women can be followed without any biochemical diagnostic testing. Severe symptoms, symptoms that do not improve after hormone therapy, or incongruent symptoms such as regular menstrual cycles with concomitant depression and fatigue, merit further investigation and consideration of a variety of related conditions.

Biochemical testing, using early follicular phase FSH measurements, should, in general, be discouraged. While these tests are useful for confirmation of limited ovarian reserve and prediction of cycle fecundity, they are of poor predictive value in determining the timing of the final menstrual period. Longitudinal measures in an individual patient lack meaning, and may further confuse both patient and practitioner, since cycle-to-cycle variation is high.

References

1. McKinlay SM. The normal menopause transition: an overview. *Maturitas* 1996;23:137–45
2. McKinlay SM, Brambilla DJ, Posner JC. The normal menopause transition. *Am J Hum Biol* 1992;4:37–46
3. Gold EB, Bromberger J, Crawford S. Factors associated with age at natural menopause in a multiethnic sample of midlife women. *Am J Epidemiol* 2001;153:865–74
4. Cooper GS, Sandler DP. Age at natural menopause and mortality. *Ann Epidemiol* 1998;8: 229–35
5. Eckholdt H, Santoro N, Luborsky J. Induced menopause in a multi-ethnic population study of the menopause. Presented at the *4th International Symposium on Women's Health and Menopause*, Washington, DC, 20–22 May 2001
6. McKinlay SM, Bifano NL, McKinlay JB. Smoking and age at menopause in women. *Ann Intern Med* 1985;103:350–6.
7. Bromberger JT, Matthews KA, Kuller LH, *et al.* Prospective study of the determinants of age at menopause. *Am J Epidemiol* 1997;145:124–33
8. Luoto R, Kaprio J, Uutela A. Age at natural menopause and sociodemographic status in Finland. *Am J Epidemiol* 1994;139:64–76
9. Harlow Bl, Signorello LB. Factors associated with early menopause. *Maturitas* 2000;35:3–9
10. Cramer DW, Xu H. Predicting age at menopause. *Maturitas* 1996;23:319–26
11. Wallace R, Sherman BM, Bean J, *et al.* Probability of menopause with increasing duration of amenorrhea in middle-aged women. *Am J Obstet Gynecol* 1979;135:1021
12. World Health Organization. *Research on the Menopause in the 1990's.* WHO Technical Report Series 866. Geneva: WHO, 1996:866
13. Brambilla DJ, McKinlay SM, Johannes CB. Defining the perimenopause for application in epidemiologic investigations. *Am J Epidemiol* 1994;140:1091–5
14. Garamszegi C, Dennerstein L, Dudley E, Guthrie JR, Ryan M, Burger H. Menopausal status: subjectively and objectively defined. *J Psychosom Obstet Gynecol* 1998;19:165–73
15. Dennerstein L, Dudley EC, Hopper JL, *et al.* A prospective, population-based study of menopausal symptoms. *Obstet Gynecol* 2000;96: 351–8
16. Campbell S, Whitehead M. Oestrogen therapy and the menopausal syndrome. *Clin Obstet Gynaecol* 1977;4:31–47
17. Kim TJ, Anasti JN, Flack MR, Kimzey LM, Defensor RA, Nelson LM. Routine endocrine screening for patients with karyotypically normal spontaneous premature ovarian failure. *Obstet Gynecol* 1997;89:777–9
18. Mendelson J, Mello NK. Diagnostic evaluation of alcohol and drug abuse problems in women. *Psychopharmacol Bull* 1998;34:279–81
19. Santoro N, Schoenbaum E, Adel T, Buono D. Substance abuse, but not HIV infection, alters reproductive hormones in midlife women. Presented at the *82nd Annual Meeting of the Endocrine Society*, Toronto, Canada, 21–24 June 2000:abstr 2324

Reproductive aging: compensated ovarian failure

2

N. A. Klein and M. R. Soules

Introduction

Aging of the human female reproductive system is a process that begins before birth and extends beyond the time of the last menstrual period. Females are born with a finite number of ovarian follicles, the majority of which will expire through a continuous process of follicle atresia. At any age, the function of the ovary and integrity of the hypothalamic–pituitary–ovarian (HPO) axis appear to be largely dependent on the number of functional ovarian follicles remaining. Loss of significant numbers of functional ovarian follicles (due to surgery, torsion, ovarian pathology such as neoplasm or endometriosis, chemotherapy, radiation, or infection) may accelerate the loss of ovarian reserve and, in severe cases, lead to premature ovarian failure.

The HPO axis is a highly integrated feedback loop which maintains regular, ovulatory menstrual cycles throughout most of the reproductive lifespan. In the early stages of reproductive aging, there is a gradual rise in follicle stimulating hormone (FSH) that is sufficient to compensate for the decreased ovarian responsiveness and loss of ovarian secretory capacity that presumably result from declining follicle numbers. Under the influence of FSH elevation, the ability to maintain regular, ovulatory cycles is usually preserved for several years in spite of advanced follicular atresia, early endocrinological changes and the onset of age-related infertility.

Ovarian follicle depletion

The physiological basis of the perimenopause and menopause can be largely attributed to changes within the ovaries. The female *in utero* at 5 months of fetal age has received her maximum endowment of primordial follicles, estimated to be about 2 million[1]. The number of follicles in the ovarian cortex gradually declines from this point onward, until only a relatively few, poorly responsive follicles remain at the time of the menopause. Relative to atresia, ovulation accounts for the loss of only a small proportion of the follicle pool; only about 500 ovulations occur in the lifespan of a normal woman. The wide range of age of menopause (mean 50 ± 8 years) implies that the initial endowment of primordial follicles and/or the rate of follicle loss is variable between individuals. How much of this variability is related to the size of the initial follicle pool or to factors affecting the rate of atresia is unknown. It appears that the physiological mechanism for this progressive loss of follicles is programmed cell death (apoptosis), influenced by a number of promoting and inhibitory factors[2]. Studies in mice raise the possibility that follicle atresia may be under pituitary control, since hypophysectomy appears to prevent it[3].

Current knowledge regarding primordial follicle depletion is based upon a combined database consisting of three published studies[1,4,5]. These studies report morphometric estimates of primordial follicle number in 103 ovarian pairs from females aged 6–55 years. Mathematical modelling has been used on this combined database to estimate the number of primordial follicles at birth (about 500 000) and to hypothesize that follicular depletion is bi-exponential with an accelerated loss occurring at about age 38[6,7].

Effect of female age on fertility

The final menstrual period occurs, on average, at about age 50. Generally, women continue to ovulate and maintain regular menstrual periods well into their mid- to late forties. Eventually, most women experience an interval of marked cycle irregularity and/or oligomenorrhea, the hallmark of the transition into menopause. The months preceding the menopause are usually associated with substantial changes in menstrual cyclicity and intermittent anovulation, and the probability of conception is remote. However, over several years prior to this time, subtle changes occur within the HPO axis, associated with a rapid and profound decline in fecundity. Although there is a gradual loss of fertility beginning as early as the mid-twenties, the rate of decline in fertility becomes much more pronounced after the age of 35[8]. Compelling evidence of this effect of female age on fertility can be derived from populations where marriage later in life is relatively common, contraception is rarely practiced and accurate birth records are maintained. In such populations, the average age of women at the time of the last pregnancy ranges between 39 and 42[9]. Menken and colleagues reported that the percentage of married women remaining childless rose steadily with age: 6% at age 20–24, 9% at age 25–29, 15% at age 30–34, 30% at age 35–39 and 64% at age 40–44[8]. This decline in fertility occurs in spite of the fact that women generally maintain regular, ovulatory menstrual cycles well into their fifth decade.

Several lines of evidence suggest that the aging oocyte is the predominant underlying cause of age-related infertility. Abnormalities present in the older oocyte include distinct differences in microtubule and chromosome placement in the second metaphase of meiosis[10,11] and higher rates of single chromatid abnormalities[12]. Embryos derived from the oocytes of older women in *in vitro* fertilization (IVF) cycles exhibit a higher frequency of aneuploidy compared with those of younger patients[13]. The incidence of spontaneous abortions, the majority of which are due to chromosomal abnormalities, also increases significantly with advanced maternal age[14]. Similarly, the rate of clinically significant cytogenetic abnormalities in live births rises from about 1/500 for women under 30, to 1/270 at age 30, 1/80 at age 35, 1/60 at age 40 and 1/20 at age 45[15]. Pregnancy and delivery rates after oocyte donation are much more strongly correlated with the age of the donor than the age of the recipient[16–19]. According to the 1999 report by the Society for Assisted Reproductive Technology and Centers for Disease Control and Prevention, no significant age-related decrease in pregnancy rates was observed in cycles of IVF using donated oocytes, where the age of the oocyte donor is relatively constant[20]. Therefore, replacing the defective oocyte with that of a younger woman appears largely, if not completely, to reverse the age-related decline in female fertility.

Changes in menstrual pattern and follicle recruitment

As women age, the average length of the menstrual cycle progressively shortens. In a classic, prospective, longitudinal study, Treloar and co-workers analyzed the menstrual records of over 2700 women, constituting 25 825 woman-years. They demonstrated that there was a progressive, age-related shortening of the menstrual cycle from a median of 28 days at age 20 to 26 days at age 40[21]. Endocrine studies of steroid and gonadotropin secretion across the menstrual cycle demonstrate that the shortened cycle length is due to a progressive shortening of the follicular phase without a significant change in luteal phase length[22,23]. The observed decrease in cycle length continues until the loss of cycle regularity (usually after the age of 43), when both average cycle length and the standard deviation begin to increase[21,24]. Ultrasound and endocrine studies of normal older ovulatory women (age 40–45) have confirmed that this shortened follicular phase is associated with development and ovulation of an apparently normal follicle in the presence of elevated circulating levels of FSH[22,25]. Metcalf has demonstrated that ovulatory frequency remains high (95%) in menstruating women aged 40–55 until the onset of oligomenorrhea, when the percentage of ovulatory cycles drops significantly[26].

Changes in gonadotropins

The most consistent endocrine finding in numerous investigations of reproductive aging has been a subtle rise in the concentration of FSH unaccompanied by a rise in luteinizing hormone (LH) (the monotropic FSH rise)[22,27–29]. FSH is elevated throughout the entire menstrual cycle (most pronounced in the early follicular phase) in older ovulatory women, initially with no differences in circulating LH concentrations[22,28]. Eventually, as aging progresses, elevated circulating levels of LH are also observed in ovulatory women, usually after age 45[28,30,31]. Although the pattern of FSH secretion remains essentially unchanged across the menstrual cycle, older ovulatory women demonstrate an earlier rise in FSH in the luteal follicular transition compared with younger women, with a significant and sustained rise being detectable prior to the onset of the menstrual period[22]. Thus, with advancing reproductive age, the early follicular phase FSH peak occurs earlier in the follicular phase, subsequently falling after ovarian inhibin and estradiol secretions increase in response to gonadotropin stimulation. Studies utilizing a gonadotropin releasing hormone (GnRH) agonist to achieve suppression of the HPO axis have confirmed that the shortened follicular phase in older subjects is associated with an earlier onset of the early follicular phase FSH peak compared with that in a younger control group[32]. Therefore, final recruitment of the dominant follicle is advanced earlier into the follicular phase, independently of hormonal influences from the preceding luteal phase. Once selected, the rate of dominant follicle growth and maturation is indistinguishable from that observed in a younger control group[32].

In an effort to determine whether the changes in gonadotropin secretion are a result of changes in GnRH pulsatility, older and younger women have been studied with frequent blood sampling in the early follicular and mid-luteal phases with conflicting results[33,34]. The studies by the present authors failed to detect a difference in either the LH pulse frequency or the amplitude, which argues against a functional change in the GnRH pulse generator as the primary explanation for the monotropic FSH rise in older women of reproductive age[33]. However, other investigators detected enhancement of the LH pulse amplitude in the late luteal phase (12 ± 1 days after the LH surge), with a more subtle increase in LH pulse frequency in both the early follicular and late luteal phases in the older (age 40–50) compared with the youngest (age 19–35) age groups. These changes were observed in spite of the fact that there were no differences in either estradiol or progesterone secretion[34]. Whether there is any age-related change in sensitivity of the hypothalamic–pituitary axis to ovarian steroid feedback inhibition is unknown. The early monotropic rise in FSH is not related to a loss of FSH bioactivity, as no difference is observed in the bioactive : immunoactive FSH ratio between women in their early twenties compared with those in their early forties[22].

Older ovulatory women demonstrate increased variability in FSH levels between menstrual cycles[35,36]. After the onset of the monotropic FSH rise, resistance to exogenous gonadotropin stimulation is observed, even in cycles where FSH levels are within the normal range[35]. Thus, in older ovulatory women, FSH elevation is definitive evidence of decreased ovarian reserve, and significant ovarian aging may be missed when sampling is performed in a single menstrual cycle. Some women with normal baseline (i.e. cycle day 3) FSH have an exaggerated FSH response to clomiphene citrate administered at a dose of 100 mg during menstrual cycle days 5–9 (clomiphene citrate challenge test, CCCT). Patients exhibiting FSH elevation on cycle day 10 of the CCCT appear to have decreased ovarian reserve, with lower cumulative pregnancy rates and decreased responsiveness to exogenous gonadotropin therapy[37]. Therefore, provocative testing such as the CCCT may identify early reproductive aging prior to the onset of a detectable early follicular phase FSH rise.

Changes in ovarian steroids

Ovulating women with regular menstrual cycles continue to have normal circulating concentrations of estradiol and progesterone after the age of 40 and the onset of the monotropic FSH rise[22,28,34]. As individual older ovulatory women near the end of this phase of regular ovulation, preovulatory estradiol levels tend to be even higher and rise earlier in the follicular phase than those seen in younger women[25,31]. Follicular fluid aspirated from the preovulatory dominant follicle from normal 40–45-year-old women contained normal steroid concentrations, with a trend toward higher follicular fluid estradiol and lower androstenedione concentrations[25]. Santoro and colleagues studied 11 cycling women aged 47 and older with daily determinations of urinary estrone conjugates and pregnanediol glucuronide. Compared with women aged 19–38, these women had elevated follicular and luteal phase estrone excretion[31]. Earlier FSH stimulation of the antral follicle cohort with earlier selection and development of the dominant follicle lead to relative increases in early follicular phase estradiol secretion[22,30]. In fact, elevated early follicular phase (day 3) estradiol has been shown to predict a poor response to controlled ovarian hyperstimulation[38], although the predictive value was lower than that of FSH elevation. Elevation of estradiol in the early follicular phase thus appears to be an independent sign of decreased ovarian reserve. The endocrine characteristics of the perimenopause have been elucidated through several small, descriptive, longitudinal studies[26,29,31,39,40]. These studies revealed that, as women approached the menopause, periods of hypoestrogenemia similar to those observed in postmenopausal women were interspersed with ovulatory and anovulatory episodes of estrogen secretion.

Progesterone secretion is generally maintained in the normal range as long as ovulatory cycles are occurring at regular intervals[22,28]. As reproductive age advances further, insufficient luteal phase progesterone secretion may be observed[30,31,39].

Changes in inhibin

Inhibin is a peptide hormone secreted by the ovary that selectively inhibits FSH. Studies of normal perimenopausal and postmenopausal women have demonstrated that total immunoreactive inhibin falls in perimenopausal women, eventually becoming undetectable after the menopause[40,41]. However, previous studies that utilized non-specific assays for total inhibin (including free α subunits and precursors) yielded conflicting results, with some (but not all) studies indicating a decline in ovarian inhibin secretion corresponding to the onset of the monotropic FSH rise. Two site-specific assays for dimeric inhibin A and B demonstrated that these two hormones exhibit distinct and different patterns across normal ovulatory menstrual cycles[42,43]. Inhibin A follows a pattern similar to that observed when total immunoreactive inhibin is measured: levels are low in the early follicular phase, rise prior to ovulation and are highest in the luteal phase[42]. In contrast, inhibin B peaks in the early follicular phase and then falls throughout the remainder of the follicular phase[42]. Inhibin B appears to be the predominant inhibin form in the follicular fluid of the developing early antral follicles, with concentrations in the follicular fluid decreasing as the dominant follicle matures. In contrast, during dominant follicle development, the follicular fluid concentrations of inhibin A rise, fall transiently after ovulation, and reach maximum levels in the luteal phase[42]. Specific assays for dimeric inhibin A and B have shown that early follicular phase secretion of inhibin B (but not inhibin A) is decreased in older ovulatory women who demonstrate a monotropic FSH rise[44–48]. One possibility is that this decrease in inhibin B concentration may be a result of fewer primordial and early antral follicles remaining in the ovaries of older women. Serum levels of inhibin B in the early follicular phase are correlated with the number of antral follicles < 5 mm as seen by transvaginal ultrasound[49]. Follicular fluid aspirated from the preovulatory dominant follicle in older ovulatory women contains normal concentrations of both inhibin A and inhibin B, indicating normal granulosa cell production of these hormones[50]. Inhibin A, the dominant inhibin of the luteal phase, appears to be unchanged in older ovulatory women in the early stages of reproductive aging[44,46]. However, similar to luteal phase progesterone secretion, inhibin A deficiency is observed as reproductive aging progresses[45,47].

Changes in activin

Activin is a member of the inhibin family of ovarian peptide hormones that selectively increases FSH secretion. Activin exists in three forms – activin A, activin B, and activin AB – and is thought to play an autocrine/paracrine role in a variety of tissues. Studies of a potential role of activin in the aging of the human female reproductive system are limited in part by difficulties in assay development. Only total activin A (both free and bound to follistatin) is readily measured in the serum by currently available assays. Most of the circulating activin A is present in a bound form, rendering the hormone biologically inactive. Although some studies suggest that serum levels of total activin A may be increased in older ovulatory women[48,51], it is unclear whether it serves an important endocrine role or is related to the monotropic FSH rise. Total serum activin A increases with age in both men and women[52]. In women, there is no age-related increase beyond the age of 50, whereas levels in men do not peak until at least age 70. Concentrations of activin A, which has multiple sites of production, do not differ between men and women under the age of 50, nor do they correlate with serum levels of FSH[52]. Follicular fluid levels of activin A are increased in older ovulatory women; however, this increase is attributable entirely to activin that is bound to follistatin and is therefore inactive[50]. In summary, the significance of activin A elevation and its relationship to reproductive aging remain poorly defined.

Other ovarian changes

Several studies have identified other evidence of generalized aging within the ovary. For example, the frequency of mitochondrial DNA mutations detected in the ovary after amplification with the polymerase chain reaction increases with advancing age[53]. The frequency of these mutations is further associated with menstrual status, occurring most frequently in postmenopausal women with amenorrhea of at least 1 year's duration[53]. The factors that lead to mitochondrial DNA mutations and corresponding effects on ovarian or oocyte function remain to be elucidated. Van Blerkom has reported an increased incidence of chromosomal abnormalities in oocytes obtained from follicles with reduced follicular fluid oxygen content, apparently as a function of blood flow as detected by ultrasound[54]. The possibility that age-related changes in ovarian perfusion lead to hypoxic intrafollicular conditions which, in turn, are related to meiotic abnormalities, is an attractive hypothesis. Whether the acceleration in follicle growth, estrogen secretion and ovulation contribute to the abnormal development of the oocytes or whether they are intrinsically abnormal is unknown.

Summary

Reproductive aging in women is closely tied to the loss of ovarian follicles through atresia. The sentinel endocrinological finding is the monotropic FSH rise, associated with a decline in ovarian inhibin B secretion. Fertility becomes significantly compromised long before overt clinical signs occur such as cycle irregularity. Compromised fertility is primarily related to oocyte dysfunction. It is unclear whether the changes in feedback signals (e.g. inhibin) from the ovary are due simply to a decrease in the number of follicles or whether there is a concomitant decline in the functional status of the follicular components due to aging. As previously noted, older ovulatory women recruit and develop a dominant follicle earlier in the cycle than younger women. Once selected, these follicles exhibit normal growth, collapse and intrafollicular steroid concentrations. Normal follicular fluid hormone concentrations suggest that the dominant follicle is fully functional in terms of its secretory capacity. These findings are indicative of a healthy follicular fluid environment in the dominant follicles of older women and may reflect a compensatory effect of FSH elevation. However, in the oocytes aspirated from these apparently normal preovulatory follicles, the alignment of chromosomes on the meiotic spindle at metaphase II is abnormal in the majority of the oocytes from older women.

Based on the information available from our studies to date we would have to conclude that, in the early stages of reproductive aging, the principal defect in the ovarian follicle resides in the oocyte, and there is no evidence that follicle development and granulosa cell function are compromised. Increased pituitary FSH secretion and improved follicular fluid steroid profiles may represent compensatory mechanisms for the poor quality of the aging oocyte. The relationships between the monotropic FSH rise, accelerated follicular atresia, a shortened follicular phase and compromised oocyte quality are yet to be defined. Further studies are therefore needed to elucidate the factors contributing to the oocyte abnormalities in women of advanced reproductive age as well as the factors that determine the rate of follicle atresia and the length of the reproductive lifespan.

References

1. Block E. Quantitative morphological investigations of the follicular system in women: variations at different ages. *Acta Anat* 1952; 14(Suppl 16):108
2. Hsueh A, Billig H, Tsafriri A. Ovarian follicle atresia: a hormonally controlled apoptotic process. *Endocr Rev* 1994;15:707–24
3. Finch C. Neuroendocrine mechanisms and aging. *Fed Proc* 1979;38:178
4. Richardson S, Senikas V, Nelson J. Follicular depletion during the menopausal transition: evidence for accelerated loss and ultimate exhaustion. *J Clin Endocrinol Metab* 1987;65: 1231–7
5. Gougeon A. Qualitative changes in medium and large antral follicles in the human ovary during the menstrual cycle. *Ann Biol Anim Biochem Biophys* 1979;19:1461–8
6. Faddy M, Gosden R, Gougeon A, Richardson S, Nelson J. Accelerated disappearance of ovarian follicles in mid-life: implications for forecasting menopause. *Hum Reprod* 1992;7:1342–6
7. Gougeon A, Ecochard R, Thalabard J. Age-related changes of the population of human ovarian follicles: increase in the disappearance rate of non-growing and early-growing follicles in aging women. *Biol Reprod* 1994;50:653–63
8. Menken J, Trussell J, Larsen U. Age and infertility. *Science* 1986;233:1389–94
9. Frank O, Bianchi PG, Campana A. The end of fertility: age, fecundity and fecundability in women. *J Biosoc Sci* 1994;26:349–68
10. Battaglia DE, Klein NA, Soules MR. Changes in centrosomal domains during meiotic maturation in the human oocyte. *Mol Hum Reprod* 1997;2:845–51
11. Battaglia D, Goodwin P, Klein N, Soules M. Influence of maternal age on meiotic spindle assembly in oocytes from naturally cycling women. *Hum Reprod* 1996;11:2217–22
12. Angell R. Aneuploidy in older women. *Hum Reprod* 1994;9:1199–201
13. Benadiva C, Kligman I, Munne S. Aneuploidy 16 in human embryos increases significantly

with maternal age. *Fertil Steril* 1996;66: 248–55

14. Stein A. A woman's age, childbearing and child rearing. *Am J Epidemiol* 1985;121:327–42

15. Hook E. Rates of chromosomal abnormalities at different maternal ages. *Obstet Gynecol* 1981; 58:282

16. Balmaceda J, Bernardini L, Ciuffardi I, *et al.* Oocyte donation in humans: a model to study the effect of age on embryo implantation rate. *Hum Reprod* 1994;9:2160–3

17. Lydic M, Liu J, Rebar R, Thomas M, Cedars M. Success of donor oocyte in *in vitro* fertilization–embryo transfer in recipients with and without premature ovarian failure. *Fertil Steril* 1996;65:98–102

18. Pantos K, Meimeti-Damianaki T, Vaxevanoglou T, Kapetanakis E. Oocyte donation in menopausal women aged over 40 years. *Hum Reprod* 1993;8:488–91

19. Sauer M, Paulson R, Ary B, Lobo R. Three hundred cycles of oocyte donation at the University of Southern California: assessing the effect of age and infertility diagnosis on pregnancy and implantation rates. *J Assist Reprod Genet* 1994;11:92–5

20. *1999 Assisted Reproductive Technology Success Rates: National Summary and Fertility Clinic Reports.* Atlanta, GA: US Department of Health and Human Services, Centers for Disease Control and Prevention, 2001

21. Treloar A, Boynton R, Behn B, Brown B. Variation of the human menstrual cycle through reproductive life. *Int J Fertil* 1967; 12:77–126

22. Klein N, Battaglia D, Fujimoto V, Davis G, Bremner W, Soules M. Reproductive aging: accelerated follicular development associated with a monotropic follicle stimulating hormone rise in normal older women. *J Clin Endocrinol Metab* 1996;81:1038–45

23. Lenton E, Landgren B, Sexton L, Harper R. Normal variation in the length of follicular phase of the menstrual cycle: effect of chronological age. *Br J Obstet Gynaecol* 1984;91:6814

24. Vollman R. The degree of variability of the length of the menstrual cycle in correlation with age of woman. *Gynaecologia* 1956;142: 310–14

25. Klein N, Battaglia D, Miller P, Branigan E, Guidice L, Soules M. Ovarian follicular development and the follicular fluid hormones and growth factors in normal women of advanced reproductive age. *J Clin Endocrinol Metab* 1996;81:1946–51

26. Metcalf M. Incidence of ovulatory cycles in women approaching the menopause. *J Biosoc Sci* 1979;11:39–48

27. Sherman B, Korenman S. Hormonal characteristics of the human menstrual cycle throughout reproductive life. *J Clin Invest* 1975;55:699–706

28. Lee S, Lenton E, Sexton L, Cooke I. The effect of age on the cyclical patterns of plasma LH, FSH, oestradiol and progesterone in women with regular menstrual cycles. *Hum Reprod* 1988;3:851–5

29. Sherman B, West J, Korenman S. The menopausal transition: analysis of LH, FSH, estradiol, and progesterone concentrations during menstrual cycles of older women. *J Clin Endocrinol Metab* 1976;42:629–36

30. Reyes F, Winter J, Faiman C. Pituitary–ovarian relationships preceding the menopause. I. A cross-sectional study of serum follicle-stimulating hormone, luteinizing hormone, prolactin, estradiol and progesterone levels. *Am J Obstet Gynecol* 1977;129:557–64

31. Santoro N, Brown J, Adel T, Skurnick J. Characterization of reproductive hormonal dynamics in the perimenopause. *J Clin Endocrinol Metab* 1996;81:1495–501

32. Harper AJ, Houmard BS, Soules MR, Klein NA. Is the short follicular phase in older women secondary to advanced or accelerated dominant follicle development? Presented at the *56th Annual Meeting of the Society for Reproductive Medicine*, Orlando, FL, October 2001

33. Klein N, Battaglia D, Clifton D, Bremner W, Soules M. The gonadotropin secretion pattern in normal women of advanced reproductive age in relation to the monotropic FSH rise. *J Soc Gynecol Invest* 1996;3:27–32

34. Reame N, Kelch R, Beitins I, Yu M, Zawacki C, Padmanabhan V. Age effects on follicle-stimulating hormone and pulsatile luteinizing hormone secretion across the menstrual cycle of premenopausal women. *J Clin Endocrinol Metab* 1996;81:1512–18

35. Scott RT, Hofman GE, Oehninger S, Muasher S. Intercycle variability of day 3 follicle-stimulating hormone levels and its effect on stimulation quality in *in vitro* fertilization. *Fertil Steril* 1990;54:297–302

36. Jain T, Lee DM, Klein NA, Soules MR. Intercycle variability of day 3 serum FSH levels in normal eumenorrheic young and older women. Presented at the *55th Annual Meeting of the American Society for Reproductive Medicine*, Toronto, Ontario, September 1999

37. Scott RT, Opsahl MS, Leonardi MR, Neall GS, Illions CH, Navot D. Life table analsis of pregnancy rates in a general infertility population related to ovarian reserve and patient age. *Hum Reprod* 1995;10:1706–10

38. Licciardi F, Liu H, Rosenwaks Z. Day 3 estradiol serum concentrations as prognosticators of ovarian stimulation response and pregnancy outcome in patients undergoing *in vitro* fertilization. *Fertil Steril* 1995;64:991–4

39. Metcalf M, Livesay J. Pregnanediol excretion in fertile women: age-related changes. *J Endocr* 1988;119:153–7

40. Hee J, MacNaughton J, Bangah M, Burger H. Perimenopausal patterns of gonadotrophins, immunoreactive inhibin, oestradiol and progesterone. *Maturitas* 1993;18:9–20

41. MacNaughton J, Banah M, McCloud P, Hee J, Burger H. Age related changes in follicle stimulating hormone, oestradiol and immunoreactive inhibin in women of reproductive age. *Clin Endocrinol* 1992;36:339. 1993;76:1340–3

42. Groome N, Illingworth P, O'Brien M, Pai R, Mather J, McNeilly A. Measurement of dimeric inhibin B throughout the human menstrual cycle. *J Clin Endocrinol Metab* 1996;81:1401–5

43. Groome N, Illingworth P, O'Brien M, *et al*. Detection of dimeric inhibin throughout the human menstrual cycle by two-site enzyme immunoassay. *Clin Endocrinol* 1994;40:717–23

44. Klein N, Illingworth P, Groome M, McNeilly A, Battaglia D, Soules M. Decreased inhibin B secretion is associated with the monotropic FSH rise in older, ovulatory women: a study of serum and follicular fluid levels of dimeric inhibin A and B in spontaneous menstrual cycles. *J Clin Endocrinol Metab* 1996;81:2742–5

45. Burger HG, Dudley EC, Hopper JL, *et al*. Prospectively measured levels of serum follicle-stimulating hormone, estradiol, and the dimeric inhibins during the menopausal transition in a population-based cohort of women. *J Clin Endocrinol Metab* 1999;84:4025–30

46. Welt CK, McNicholl DJ, Taylor AE, Hall JE. Female reproductive aging is marked by decreased secretion of dimeric inhibin. *J Clin Endocrinol Metab* 1999;84:105–11

47. Danforth DR, Arbogast LK, Mroueh J, *et al*. Dimeric inhibin: a direct marker of ovarian aging. *Fertil Steril* 1998;70:119–23

48. Reame NE, Wyman TL, Phillips DJ, de Kretser DM, Padmanabhan V. Net increase in stimulatory input resulting from a decrease in inhibin B and an increase in activin A may contribute in part to the rise in follicular phase follicle-stimulating hormone of aging cycling women. *J Clin Endocrinol Metab* 1998;83:3302–7

49. Tinkanen H, Blauer M, Laippala P, Tuohimaa P, Kujansuu E. Correlation between serum inhibin B and other indicators of the ovarian function. *Eur J Obstet Gynecol Reprod Biol* 2001;94:109–13

50. Klein NA, Battaglia DE, Woodruff TK, *et al*. Ovarian follicular concentrations of activin, follistatin, inhibin, insulin-like growth factor I (IGF-I), IGF-II, IGF-binding protein-2 (IGFBP-2), IGFBP-3, and vascular endothelial growth factor in spontaneous menstrual cycles of normal women of advanced reproductive age. *J Clin Endocrinol Metab* 2000;85:4520–5

51. Santoro N, Tovaghgol A, Skurnick JH. Decreased inhibin tone and decreased activin A secretion characterize reproductive aging in women. *Fertil Steril* 1999;71:658–62

52. Loria P, Petralglia F, Concari M, *et al*. Influence of age and sex on serum concentrations of total dimeric activin A. *Eur J Endocrinol* 1998;139:469–71

53. Suganuma N, Kitagawa T, Nawa A, Tomoda Y. Human ovarian aging and mitochondrial DNA deletion. *Horm Res* 1993;39:16–21

54. Van Blerkom J. The influence of intrinsic and extrinsic factors on the developmental potential and chromosomal normality of the human oocyte. *J Soc Gynecol Invest* 1996;3:3–11

Hormonal patterns in the later menopause transition

3

H. Burger and N. Santoro

Introduction

The menopausal transition is a process of indeterminate length that encompasses the later reproductive years of a woman's life up to and including the final menstrual period. The final menstrual period defines the attainment of menopause retrospectively, and is achieved when a woman has had at least 12 consecutive months of amenorrhea[1]. Prior to the final menstrual period, a series of changes in cycles and hormones appears to occur. These changes have been partially characterized. This chapter focuses on the known changes that occur as women traverse the menopause, and some caveats are necessary at the outset. First, the existing database of hormones and patterns of change is confined almost exclusively to women who were menstruating regularly during their peak reproductive years. Little is known about the hormonal experience of hysterectomized women, and non-Caucasian women have been under-represented in most studies to date.

In characterizing the hormonal changes of the menopausal transition, one is attempting to chronicle ovarian events in the peripheral circulation. This is sometimes a frustrating enterprise, as there are no factors elaborated by the reserve follicle pool known to circulate, and the reserve follicle pool is, of course, the item of interest and the underlying reason for menopause in the first place. The discovery of a stable marker that could provide information about the numbers of remaining ovarian follicles would be of enormous benefit to this field. However, in the absence of such a marker, we are forced to attempt to piece together the events of the ovarian process based on the use of other pituitary and ovarian hormones produced by follicles in the later stages of growth and differentiation.

Definitions

Most available definitions of the menopause transition are based on menstrual patterns reported by women, and not on specific hormonal changes. Women are judged to have entered the menopause transition when they experience a detectable change in the regularity of their cycles, or skip a menstrual period[2]. Because the changes in hormones that accompany this detectable menstrual cycle change are not abrupt, but rather represent a gradual process, at present there is no measurable hormonal parameter that could be used to assist the diagnosis of entry into the menopause transition. The duration of this phase is probably variable, with longer transitions associated with earlier age at onset of this change, and shorter transitions associated with later age at onset[3].

The 'late' menopause transition is attained when a woman has experienced 3–11 months of amenorrhea. This phase is more predictive of attainment of the final menstrual period, with 95% of women becoming menopausal within 4 years[4]. Examination of menstrual cycle patterns again provides some prognostic insight – when women attain an average intermenstrual interval of more than 42 days, they are far more likely to become menopausal[5].

Hormonal patterns associated with the stages of the menopause transition

Several small and large studies have provided a series of snapshots of the process of the menopause transition. In general, the smaller studies have contained more detail and information about individual cycles or even strings of cycles, while the larger studies have included longitudinal sampling on an annual basis to characterize broader, within-woman changes.

Initial characterization of the cycles of women who are approaching menopause was provided by Sherman and associates in 1976[6]. In this study, the cycles of women aged over 45 years were examined using daily blood sampling for varying lengths of time. These investigators observed a monotropic rise in follicle stimulating hormone (FSH), variability in the proportion of ovulatory cycles and fluctuations in estradiol and progesterone production. They hypothesized that the monotropic rise in FSH that accompanied the menopause transition was due to loss of inhibin production by the ovary, a conjecture that has since been confirmed. These studies were followed by a series of urinary sampling studies by Metcalf and colleagues. In a series of studies of New Zealand women, Metcalf and colleagues documented that the proportions of ovulatory cycles decreased as women progressed through the menopause transition[7], confirmed the monotropic FSH rise in urinary samples[8] and reported that the sentinel event associated with attainment of the final menstrual period was that progesterone production appeared to cease permanently thereafter[9]. Using weekly or biweekly urinary sampling, Metcalf and colleagues did not report luteal dysfunction associated with the menopause transition, but the sampling paradigm may have been insufficient to detect this cycle change. Others have reported luteal insufficiency in the cycles of women in the menopause transition[10–12].

When annual sampling has been used in large populations of women, a progressive rise in FSH is observed throughout the menopause transition[13,14]. This is accompanied by a decrease in estradiol, although the decline in estradiol is not obvious until women get very close to their final menstrual period[13]. Early follicular phase sampling has demonstrated a progressive decline in inhibin B, but this predictor of the final menstrual period does not appear to be superior to FSH[15]. Inhibin A is also observed to decline in the follicular phase of the cycle, but this decline is not noted until the later stages of the menopause transition[16].

More recent studies of the cycles of women traversing the menopause transition have demonstrated a variety of findings. Taken together, with an attempt to place these changes in chronological order, the following series of changes appears to occur. First, before women notice a change in their menstrual cyclicity, they experience decreased ovarian reserve and sporadic increases in early follicular phase FSH[17,18]. The length of the follicular phase may decrease, as has been shown in some epidemiological studies[19]. These cycles may demonstrate few additional endocrine alterations. Inhibin B may also serve as a surrogate marker for decreased ovarian reserve[15,20]. As women progress further into more overt menstrual cycle disruption that is detectable, they experience further extremes in their reproductive hormonal patterns. FSH may increase further, and this rise is probably more consistent and lasts for more of the cycle. Inhibin B is clearly decreased[15,21–23], and luteal dysfunction, short luteal phases and decreased luteal progesterone production may occur. Inhibin A may decrease in the late follicular and luteal phases of the cycle[22,23], and increased activin A has been observed[21,22], although the endocrine role of activin A is not yet understood. As cycles become more scarce, and women enter the later stage of the menopause transition, anovulation and prolonged episodes of hypoestrogenemia coexist with lengthy elevations of FSH. In the first year after the final menstrual period (while a woman is anticipating defining herself as menopausal), variable amounts of estrogen production may be observed, although they are not accompanied by ovulation[9].

Other hormonal changes

Adrenal androgens decrease with age, with the sharpest decline occurring between the ages of 20 and 40[24,25]. There is no evidence that this age-related decline is either accelerated or ameliorated by the menopause transition. Ovarian androgens, testosterone and androstenedione, are known to decrease over the reproductive years, with the most pronounced decline occurring prior to the final menstrual period[14,26]. Modest changes in sex hormone binding globulin (SHBG) have also been reported, but there is not a dramatic decrease in the free androgen index, and in some studies this has been reported to rise at the end of the menopause transition[26,27].

Central nervous system hormone pattern changes

Pulsatile release of gonadotropin releasing hormone (GnRH) drives the production of luteinizing hormone (LH), and there is evidence that the LH pulse frequency changes with reproductive aging. Reame and co-workers[21] observed an increased luteal phase LH pulse frequency in women in their forties. Early follicular phase LH pulsations have not been noted to differ between older and younger reproductive-aged women in two studies[28,29]. However, Matt and colleagues have reported decreased LH pulse amplitude and frequency in the mid-follicular phase of the cycle of older reproductive-aged women[30]. This finding implies that women have some evidence of enhanced sensitivity to the negative feedback of mid-follicular estradiol on their hypothalamic–pituitary axis, or that mid-follicular phase estradiol is elevated in women at some point in their menopause transition. There is support for both of these notions.

Anovulatory cycles become more common in women as they progress through the menopause transition. In some of these cycles, there is evidence of massive estrogen production, in which there is no progesterone production[11,12]. These cycles, seen in many normal women, had previously been attributed to women with dysfunctional uterine bleeding[31]. However, more recent data suggest that failure to respond to an estradiol challenge with an LH surge is a relatively common finding in women who have entered the menopause transition[32,33]. As the transition progresses further, and the ovary can no longer compensate, anovulation and prolonged amenorrhea ensue. The pathophysiology and mechanisms of this physiological, age-related anovulation remain to be elucidated.

Conclusions

Taken together, the available evidence permits us to create the following chronology. The follicle cohort shrinks throughout life. Concomitantly, FSH rises. These concurrent events reach a critical level during a woman's reproductive life, at which she begins to experience a marked decline in fertility but has no other noticeable evidence of cycle dysfunction. As the process progresses further, and the follicle cohort shrinks to a certain threshold, cycle changes begin to occur that may or may not be noticeable but become measurable. Inhibin B declines, reflective of the decreased follicle pool, and FSH rises in reaction to the loss of inhibin restraint. Since, at this point, the ovary still contains sufficient responsive follicles, the rise in FSH causes noticeable cycle changes, such as a shortened follicular phase, increased early follicular, and, in some studies, whole cycle estrogen, and possibly luteal dysfunction. This stage may be conceptualized as 'compensated failure'. A 'threshold' of inhibin B (or other peptides for which inhibin B is a marker) is reached which initiates a critical level of 'decompensation'. This phenomenon may be due to an intolerable 'compression' of the follicular phase, an initiation of inappropriate periovulatory events, or serial cycles with short follicular phases and high FSH that create hypothalamic–pituitary axis dysfunction.

At some point, currently undefined endocrinologically, the follicle pool decreases to an intolerably low level and FSH rises further and more consistently. The ovary finally fails to recruit follicles, and a woman skips a cycle and enters the menopause transition. During the menopause transition, numerous mitigating factors (such as age and smoking, to name two) may affect the ultimate time to menopause. Variable cycle function occurs, and fertility, though possible, is extremely unlikely. Finally, the follicle pool available for recruitment is essentially exhausted, and the final menstrual period is attained.

References

1. Wallace R, Sherman BM, Bean J, *et al*. Probability of menopause with increasing duration of amenorrhea in middle-aged women. *Am J Obstet Gynecol* 1979;135:1021
2. Brambilla DJ, McKinlay SM, Johannes CB. Defining the perimenopause for application in epidemiologic investigations. *Am J Epidemiol* 1994;140:1091–5
3. McKinlay SM. The normal menopause transition: an overview. *Maturitas* 1996;23:137–45
4. Garamszegi C, Dennerstein L, Dudley E, Guthrie JR, Ryan M, Burger H. Menopausal status: subjectively and objectively defined. *J Psychosom Obstet Gynecol* 1998;19:165–73
5. Taffe J, Dennerstein L. Menstrual patterns leading to the final menstrual period. *Menopause* 2002;9:32–40
6. Sherman BM, West JH, Korenman SG. The menopausal transition: analysis of LH, FSH, estradiol and progesterone concentration during menstrual cycles of older women. *J Clin Endocrinol Metab* 1976;42:629–36
7. Metcalf M. Incidence of ovulatory cycles in women approaching the menopause. *J Biosoc Sci* 1979;11:39–48
8. Metcalf MG, Donald RA, Livesey JH. Pituitary ovarian function in normal women during the menopausal transition. *Clin Endocrinol* 1981;14:234–55
9. Metcalf MG, Donald RA, Livesey JH. Pituitary–ovarian function before, during and after the menopause: a longitudinal study. *Clin Endocrinol (Oxf)* 1982;17:489–94
10. Reyes F, Winter J, Faiman C. Pituitary–ovarian relationships preceding the menopause. I. A cross-sectional study of serum follicle-stimulating hormone, luteinizing hormone, prolactin, estradiol and progesterone levels. *Am J Obstet Gynecol* 1977;129:557–64
11. Santoro N, Brown JR, Adel T, Skurnick JH. Characterization of reproductive hormonal dynamics in the perimenopause. *J Clin Endocrinol Metab* 1996;81:1495–501
12. Shideler SE, De Vane GW, Kaira PS, Benirschke K, Lasley BL. Ovarian–pituitary hormone interactions during the perimenopause. *Maturitas* 1989;11:331–9
13. Burger HG, Dudley EC, Hopper JL, *et al*. The endocrinology of the menopausal transition: a cross-sectional study of a population-based sample. *J Clin Endocrinol Metab* 1995;80:3537–45
14. Rannevik G, Caristrom K, Jeppsson S, *et al*. A prospective, long-term study in women from premenopause to postmenopause: changing profiles of gonadotropins, oestrogens and androgens. *Maturitas* 1986;8:297–307
15. Burger HG, Dudley EC, Hopper JL, *et al*. Prospectively measured levels of serum follicle-stimulating hormone, estradiol, and the dimeric inhibins during the menopausal transition in a population-based cohort of women. *J Clin Endocrinol Metab* 1999;84:4025–30
16. Burger HG. Perimenopausal changes in FSH, the inhibins and the circulating steroid hormone milieu. In Lobo RA, Kelsey J, Marcus R, eds. *Menopause: Biology and Pathobiology*. San Diego: Academic Press, 2000:147–55
17. Faddy MJ, Gosden RG, Gougeon A, Richardson SJ, Nelson JF. Accelerated disappearance of ovarian follicles in mid-life: implications for forecasting menopause. *Hum Reprod* 1992;7:1342–6
18. Klein NA, Battaglia D, Fujimoto V, Davis G, Bremner W, Soules M. Reproductive aging: accelerated follicular development associated with a monotropic follicle stimulating hormone rise in normal or older women. *J Clin Endocrinol Metab* 1996;81:1038–45
19. Lee SJ, Lenton EA, Sexton L, Cooke ID. The effect of age on the cyclical patterns of plasma LH, FSH, oestradiol and progesterone in women with regular menstrual cycles. *Hum Reprod* 1988;3:851–5
20. Klein NA, Illingworth PJ, Groome NP, McNeilly AS, Battaglia DE, Soules MR.

Decreased inhibin B is associated with the monotropic FSH rise in older, ovulatory women: a study of serum and follicular fluid levels of dimeric inhibin A and B in spontaneous menstrual cycles. *J Clin Endocrinol Metab* 1996;81:2742–5

21. Reame NE, Wyman TL, Phillips DJ, de Kretser DM, Padmanabhan V. Net increase in stimulatory input resulting from a decrease in inhibin B and an increase in activin A may contribute in part to the rise in follicular phase follicle-stimulating hormone of aging, cycling women. *J Clin Endocrinol Metab* 1998;83:3302–7

22. Santoro N, Adel T, Skurnick JH. Decreased inhibin tone and increased activin A secretion characterize reproductive aging in women. *Fertil Steril* 1999;71:658–62

23. Welt CK, McNicholl DJ, Taylor AE, Hall JE. Female reproductive aging is marked by decreased secretion of dimeric inhibin. *J Clin Endocrinol Metab* 1999;84:105–11

24. Labrie F, Belanger A, Cusan L, *et al*. Marked decline in serum concentrations of adrenal C19 sex steroid precursors and androgen metabolites during aging. *J Clin Endocrinol Metab* 1997;82:2396–402

25. Orentreich N, Brind JL, Riser RL, *et al*. Age changes and sex differences in serum dehydroepiandrosterone sulfate concentrations throughout adulthood. *J Clin Endocrinol Metab* 1984;59:551–5

26. Burger HG, Dudley ED, Cui J, *et al*. A prospective, longitudinal study of serum testosterone, dehydroepiandrosterone, androstenedione and sex hormone-binding globulin levels through the menopause transition. *J Clin Endocrinol Metab* 2000;85:2832–8

27. Longcope C, Franz C, Morello C, *et al*. Steroid and gonadotropin levels in women during the perimenopausal years. *Maturitas* 1986;8:189–96

28. Klein NA, Battaglia DE, Clifton DK, Bremner WJ, Soules MR. The gonadotropin secretion pattern in normal women of advanced reproductive age in relation to the monotropic rise of FSH. *J Soc Gynecol Invest* 1996;3:27–32

29. Wilshire GB, Loughlin JS, Brown JR, Adel TE, Santoro N. Diminished function of the somatotrophic axis in older reproductive-aged women. *J Clin Endocrinol Metab* 1995;80:608–13

30. Matt DW, Kauma SW, Pincus SM. Characteristics of luteinizing hormone secretion in younger versus older premenopausal women. *Am J Obstet Gynecol* 1998;178:504–10

31. Van Look PFA, Lothian H, Hunter WM, Michie EA, Baird DT. Hypothalamic–pituitary–ovarian function in perimenopausal women. *Clin Endocrinol* 1977;7:13–31

32. Cano A, Gimeno F, Fuente T, Parrilla JJ, Abad L. The positive feedback of estradiol on gonadotropin secretion in women with dysfunctional uterine bleeding. *Eur J Obstet Gynecol Reprod Biol* 1986;22:353–8

33. Park SJ, Goldsmith LT, Reinert A, Skurnick JH, Weiss GE. Perimenopausal women are deficient in an estrogen positive feedback on LH secretion mechanism. Presented at the *82nd Annual Meeting of the Endocrine Society*, Toronto, Canada, 21–24 June 2000:abstr 248

Body composition changes in midlife

4

C. K. Sites

Introduction

The menopause transition is associated with metabolic and cardiovascular changes that have long-lasting effects on health status. The mechanisms underlying the increase in metabolic and cardiovascular risk after menopause are unknown, but could involve changes in body composition, energy expenditure, resting metabolic rate, or physical activity during the menopause transition. This review focuses on changes in energy expenditure and body composition that occur with menopause, and examines the effect of hormone replacement therapy on these changes.

Energy expenditure

One possible mechanism behind the increase in metabolic and cardiovascular risk with menopause could involve decreased energy expenditure with the menopause transition. Body fat is gained during periods of energy imbalance, when more energy is consumed than is expended. If long-lasting, this energy imbalance could lead to increased body fat, with resulting increases in metabolic and cardiovascular risk. It appears that post-menopausal women have greater total body fat than premenopausal women of similar age[1].

Energy intake is periodic, whereas daily energy expenditure is continuous. Total daily energy expenditure includes the following components: resting metabolic rate (RMR), the thermic effect of a meal, and physical activity daily energy expenditure (Figure 1). Representing the largest portion of total daily

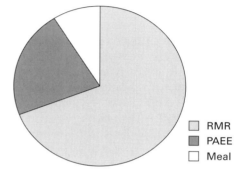

Figure 1 Total daily energy expenditure is composed of resting metabolic rate (RMR), 60–75%; physical activity daily energy expenditure (PAEE), 10–30%; and the thermic effect of a meal (Meal), 10%

energy expenditure (60–75%), resting metabolic rate is the energy expended for the maintenance of physiologic homeostasis[2]. The thermic effect of a meal is the increase in energy associated with meal ingestion, and represents approximately 10% of total daily energy expenditure. The most variable part of daily energy expenditure is the effect of physical activity. In addition to traditional exercise, this component includes such daily activities as shivering and fidgeting. Approximately 10–30% of daily caloric expenditure is composed of physical activity. It is currently unknown how these components change with the menopause transition and how they may relate to changes in body composition and cardiovascular risk. Furthermore, it is unclear if these changes surpass those of the normal aging process, or if hormone replacement therapy affects them. Ongoing, longitudinal studies of premenopausal women during the menopausal transition, as well as studies of postmenopausal women on hormone replacement therapy, will provide answers to these questions in the future.

Resting metabolic rate

Since resting metabolic rate makes the largest contribution to total daily energy expenditure, changes in this parameter have great potential to affect the regulation of body weight during menopause. Cross-sectional studies have suggested that menopause may accelerate the decline in resting metabolic rate[3,4]. Although no changes in resting metabolic rate were found in women up to age 48 years, a decrease of 4–5% per decade was noted after this point[3]. During the menopause transition, this decrease could account for an increase in total body fat of 3–4 kg. These cross-sectional studies suggest that menopause may be related to lower resting energy expenditure.

The effect of natural menopause on energy expenditure was reported in a longitudinal study[5]. In this study, women who experienced menopause were compared with women of similar age who remained premenopausal. In women who became postmenopausal, resting metabolic rate decreased by approximately 420 kJ/day, compared with no significant change in women who remained premenopausal. In addition, fat-free (lean) mass decreased by 3 kg in the postmenopausal group only. Since fat-free mass is the main determinant of resting metabolic rate, it is possible that the decrease in fat-free mass contributed to the decline in resting metabolic rate. This longitudinal study suggests that the menopause transition accelerates the decline in resting metabolic rate beyond that of aging itself.

Physical activity and food intake

Although physical activity represents a smaller portion of total daily energy expenditure than does resting metabolic rate, it is more variable, and can be influenced by behavioral changes during menopause. Both consistent increases or decreases in physical activity could impact on body weight. It is unclear whether changes in menopausal status affect physical activity. In a cross-sectional study of older women, decreased physical activity contributed to the decrease in metabolic rate; however, menopause *per se* did not contribute independently to this finding[4]. However, in a longitudinal study, physical activity declined with menopause[5]. In this study, premenopausal and postmenopausal women had similar levels of fitness as measured by peak VO_2, but postmenopausal women reported less leisure time physical activity on a questionnaire (−531 kJ/day). A decline in reported physical activity in addition to a reduction in resting metabolic rate could account for an increase in body fat and decrease in lean body mass during the menopause transition. This outcome would be especially likely without a simultaneous decrease in food intake.

The effect of menopause on food intake is not clear and is subject to behavioral modification. Hormone replacement therapy does not appear to affect food intake in postmenopausal women[6]. In a recent study of postmenopausal women classified as long-term restrained or unrestrained eaters, restrained eaters had lower physical activity energy expenditure than the unrestrained eaters, despite similar total daily energy expenditure between groups[7]. This lower level of physical activity energy expenditure in restrained eaters compared with unrestrained eaters was apparently due to reduced non-exercise activity thermogenesis (e.g. fidgeting and shivering) in the restrained eater group. Future studies should address the issue of food intake as a function of menopausal status.

Body fat accumulation and distribution

With decreased energy expenditure during the menopause transition, women are likely to experience an accumulation of body fat.

Several studies suggest that women increase body weight with age[8], and that these changes may be increased further as a result of the menopause[9-12]. Others report no increase in weight due to menopause *per se*[13]. Studies that report changes in weight due to menopause are of interest to women, but do not reflect the variety of body compartments which are important to health (fat mass, muscle mass, bone mass, and body water). Changes in body fat distribution that occur with aging may begin near the time of menopause and may reflect health status later[10].

In a cross-sectional study of 53 non-obese late premenopausal women and 28 early non-obese postmenopausal women of similar age, we found that total body fat was 28% higher in postmenopausal compared with premenopausal women[1]. Furthermore, postmenopausal women had 49% more intra-abdominal fat and 22% greater subcutaneous abdominal fat than premenopausal women. The menopause-related difference in intra-abdominal fat persisted after statistical adjustment for total body fat and age, although the subcutaneous abdominal fat difference did not. These data suggest that the early postmenopausal state is associated with a preferential increase in intra-abdominal fat which is independent of age and total body fat.

What is the significance of an increase in central body fat, particularly intra-abdominal fat? The accumulation of central or intra-abdominal fat is strongly correlated to metabolic complications that result in increased risk for diabetes and heart disease[14,15]. Particularly in normal weight postmenopausal women, central fat is more related to elevated insulin and triglycerides than is body mass index[16]. Mechanisms explaining how intra-abdominal fat affects metabolic disease remain unclear. It has been shown that adipose tissue located in the abdominal cavity is very lipolytic, releasing large amounts of free fatty acids in the circulation[17]. High levels of free fatty acids in the portal vein may increase the secretion of triglyceride-rich lipoproteins and apolipoprotein B production by the liver[18]. Therefore, intra-abdominal fat could

affect cardiovascular risk through adverse changes in the lipid profile.

Circulating markers of inflammation have also recently been shown to be important and are independent risk factors for cardiovascular disease in women at midlife[19]. In this population, high sensitivity C-reactive protein (CRP) and interleukin 6 (IL-6) are associated with increased cardiovascular events. It has also been shown that human fat produces the inflammation marker tumor necrosis factor-alpha (TNF-α)[20]. The link between circulating markers of inflammation and cardiovascular disease is not well understood, but could involve the production of inflammation markers by fat. We have recently reported that postmenopausal status is characterized by higher circulating TNF-α concentrations compared with premenopausal status[21]. In this study, CRP was positively related to intra-abdominal fat in postmenopausal but not in premenopausal women. Taken together, these studies suggest that menopausal status affects plasma levels of inflammation markers and their relationship to intra-abdominal fat, which could partly explain the association between inflammation markers and cardiovascular risk in postmenopausal women.

The most commonly used method to estimate the accumulation of fat in the abdominal region has been the ratio of the waist circumference to hip circumference (waist-to-hip ratio). Waist circumference has been suggested as a better estimate of intra-abdominal fat than waist-to-hip ratio[22]. In some studies, dual photon X-ray absorptiometry (DXA) has also been used to measure the proportion of trunk fat, which can be used as a surrogate for abdominal fat[23]. Although DXA may be more precise than waist-to-hip ratio, it does not provide any information on the amount of fat located inside the abdominal cavity compared with the subcutaneous abdominal fat. Computer assisted tomography (CT) and magnetic resonance imaging (MRI) have been employed in studies more recently to measure precisely intra-abdominal and subcutaneous abdominal fat[24,25]. With these techniques, a single scan is performed at the L4–L5

Table 1 Studies of hormone replacement therapy (HRT) and body composition

Study	n	Design	HRT regimen	Results
Haarbo et al.[26] (1991)	62	randomized, placebo-controlled	E_2V + CPA, E_2V + LVG vs. placebo	treatment prevents the increase in abdominal fat found with placebo (DPA/DXA used)
Aloia et al.[9] (1995)	94	randomized, placebo-controlled	CEE + MP vs. placebo	treatment has no effect on leg-to-trunk fat ratio (DPA)
Reubinoff et al.[6] (1995)	63	non-randomized	CEE + CPA vs. no treatment	treatment prevents the increase in abdominal adiposity (WHR) found with no treatment
Gambacciani et al.[27] (1997)	27	non-randomized	E_2V + CPA vs. control	treatment prevents the increase in abdominal adiposity (DXA) found with control group
Espeland et al.[28] (1997)	875	randomized, placebo-controlled	CEE, CEE + MPA, CEE + MP vs. placebo	treatment prevents the increase in waist circumference found in placebo group
Davis et al.[33] (2000)	33	randomized	E_2 implant vs. E_2 + T implant	treatment with E_2 caused reduced abdominal circumference compared with E_2 + T treatment
Gambacciani et al.[29] (2001)	31	non-randomized	E_2 + CPA vs. control	treatment prevents the increase in abdominal adiposity (DXA) found with control group, but causes an increase in leg fat
Walker et al.[31] (2001)	30	randomized, placebo-controlled	E_2 + norethisterone acetate	treatment did not affect abdominal adiposity (DXA) compared with placebo
Anderson et al.[32] (2001)	33	non-randomized; younger vs. older postmenopausal women	transdermal E_2 + vaginal P	short-term treatment did not affect abdominal adiposity (WHR) in older or younger women
Sites et al.[30] (2001)	45	cross-sectional; obese women	E_2 or CEE + MPA	HRT users had less intra-abdominal fat (CT) compared with non-users after adjustment for total fat
Dobs et al.[34] (2002)	40	randomized	CEE vs. CEE + methyltestosterone	treatment with CEE + methyl-testosterone increased total lean body mass and weight without increasing trunk fat (DXA) compared with CEE alone

E_2V, estradiol valerate; LVG, levonorgestrel; CEE, conjugated estrogens; MP, micronized progesterone; CPA, cyproterone acetate; DPA, dual photon absorptiometry; DXA, dual X-ray absorptiometry; MPA, medroxyprogesterone acetate; T, testosterone; E_2, estradiol; WHR, waist-to-hip ratio; CT, computed tomography scan

vertebral disk space, and the selected fat compartment can be measured. A single scan has been shown to accurately represent the entire intra-abdominal fat volume. At this time, CT and MRI remain more important in research studies than in actual office practice to measure fat distribution. However, links between intra-abdominal fat and measurable cardiovascular risk factors, such as lipids, homocysteine, insulin and glucose, may become important in counselling postmenopausal women about cardiovascular risk.

Hormone replacement therapy

Hormone replacement therapy (HRT) has been suggested as a treatment for early postmenopausal women to prevent the increase in central body fat (Table 1). In trials employing various estrogens and progestins over 1–5 years, hormone replacement appeared to be beneficial in the majority of studies[6,26–29]. In these studies, body fat was measured by anthropometry or DXA. In general, a 6.5% increase in central fat was noted in control groups, while small or no changes were noted in HRT treatment groups[6,26,28]. In one cross-sectional study of obese women where CT was used to measure intra-abdominal fat, HRT users had less intra-abdominal fat than non-users[30].

In several studies, no effect of combined estrogen plus progestin on body fat distribution was noted[9,31,32]. In two of these studies, natural progesterone (oral micronized progesterone or vaginal progesterone) was employed[9,32]. It is difficult to attribute differences in outcomes to the progestin, however, since Espeland found no differences in waist circumference with various progestins[28]. Few studies have examined the effect of added testosterone to estrogen replacement, and those that have been carried out have found varied results[33,34].

In summary, the majority of trials employing anthropometric methods, dual photon absorptiometry (DPA) or DXA found that combined estrogen plus progestin regimens reduced central adiposity in postmenopausal women compared with control or placebo. There is very little information available with regard to the effect of testosterone replacement on body composition and body fat distribution in postmenopausal women. Ongoing trials employing CT will provide additional information in the future with regard to the effect of HRT on intra-abdominal fat.

Conclusions

Energy expenditure declines with both aging and menopause. It is presently unclear if the menopause transition accelerates this decline more than the aging process itself. The decrease in energy expenditure during menopause may be due to a reduction in resting metabolic rate, along with a decrease in physical activity energy expenditure. If not accompanied by a decrease in food intake, these changes may result in increased total body fat. Lean body mass also declines, contributing to the decreased resting metabolic rate. Body composition may change during the menopause transition, resulting in more central fat. Whether this central fat accumulation is more intra-abdominal (which could lead to more serious metabolic consequences) or subcutaneous remains to be determined.

Combined estrogen plus progestin hormone replacement therapy may reduce central fat. No particular regimen appears superior to others in this regard. Ongoing randomized trials will provide more information on the possible health benefits of hormone replacement therapy to reduce intra-abdominal fat and risk for metabolic and cardiovascular disease.

Acknowledgement

This work was supported by NIH grants AG15121 and M01RR1093252.

References

1. Toth MJ, Tchernof A, Sites CK, Poehlman ET. Effect of menopausal status on body composition and abdominal fat distribution. *Int J Obes Relat Metab Disord* 2000;24:226–31
2. Toth MJ. Energy expenditure in wasting diseases: current concepts and measurement techniques. *Curr Opin Clin Nutr Metab Care* 1999;2:445–51
3. Poehlman ET, Goran MI, Gardner AW, *et al.* Metabolic determinants of the decline in resting metabolic rate in aging females. *Am J Physiol* 1993;264:E450–5

4. Arciero PJ, Goran MI, Poehlman ET. Resting metabolic rate is lower in females compared to males. *J Appl Physiol* 1993;75:2514–20

5. Poehlman ET, Toth MJ, Gardner AW. Changes in energy balance and body composition at the menopause: a controlled longitudinal study. *Ann Intern Med* 1995;123:673–5

6. Reubinoff BE, Wurtman J, Rojansky N, *et al*. Effects of hormone replacement therapy on weight, body composition, fat distribution, and food intake in early postmenopausal women: a prospective study. *Fertil Steril* 1995;64:963–8

7. Bathalon GP, Hays NP, McCrory MA, *et al*. The energy expenditure of postmenopausal women classified as restrained or unrestrained eaters. *Eur J Clin Nutr* 2001;55:1059–67

8. Poehlman ET, Toth MJ, Bunyanrd LB, *et al*. Physiological predictors of increasing total and central adiposity in aging men and women. *Arch Intern Med* 1995;155:2443–88

9. Aloia JF, McGowan GM, Vaswani AN, Ross P, Cohn SH. Relationship of menopause to skeletal and muscle mass. *Am J Clin Nutr* 1991; 53:1378–83

10. Enzi G, Gasparo M, Biondetti PR, Fiore D, Semisa M, Zurlo F. Subcutaneous and visceral fat distribution according to sex, age, and overweight, evaluated by computed tomography. *Am J Clin Nutr* 1986;44:739–46

11. den Tonkelaar I, Seidell JC, van Noord PA, Baanders-van Halewijn EA, Ouwehand IJ. Fat distribution in relation to age, degree of obesity, smoking habits, parity and estrogen use: a cross-sectional study in 11 825 Dutch women participating in the DOM-project. *Int J Obes* 1990;14:753–61

12. Pasquali R, Vicennati V, Bertazzo D, *et al*. Determinants of sex hormone-binding globulin blood concentration in premenopausal and postmenopausal women with different estrogen status. *Metabolism* 1997;46:5–9

13. Wing RR, Matthews KA, Kuller LH, Meilahn EN, Plantinga PL. Weight gain at the time of menopause. *Arch Intern Med* 1991;151:97–102

14. Despres JP, Moorjani S, Lupien PJ, Tremblay A, Nadeau A, Bouchard C. Regional distribution of body fat, plasma lipoproteins and cardiovascular disease. *Arteriosclerosis* 1990;10: 497–511

15. Hernandez-Ono A, Monter-Carreola G, Zamora-Gonzalez J, *et al*. Association of visceral fat with coronary risk factors in a population-based sample of postmenopausal women. *Int J Obes Relat Metab Disord* 2002;26:33–9

16. Van Pelt RE, Evans EM, Schechtman KB, Ehsani AA, Kohrt WM. Waist circumference vs. body mass index for prediction of disease risk in postmenopausal women. *Int J Obes Relat Metab Disord* 2001;25:1183–8

17. Mauriege P, Prud'homme D, Lemieux S, Tremblay A, Despres JP. Regional differences in adipose tissue lipolysis from lean and obese women: existence of postreceptor alterations. *Am J Physiol* 1995;269:E341–50

18. Bjortorp P. Portal adipose tissue as a generator of risk factors for cardiovascular disease and diabetes. *Arterioscler Thromb* 1990;10:493–6

19. Ridker PM, Hennekens CH, Buring JE, Rifai N. C-reactive protein and other markers of inflammation in the prediction of cardiovascular disease in women. *N Engl J Med* 2000;342: 836–43

20. Hotamisligil GS, Arner P, Caro JF, Atkinson RL, Spiegelman BM. Increased adipose tissue expression of tumor necrosis factor-α in human obesity and insulin resistance. *J Clin Invest* 1995;95:2409–15

21. Sites CK, Toth MJ, Cushman M, *et al*. Menopause-related differences in inflammation markers and their relationship to body fat distribution and insulin-stimulated glucose disposal. *Fertil Steril* 2002;77:128–35

22. Pouliot MC, Despres JP, Lemieux S, *et al*. Waist circumference and abdominal sagittal diameter: best simple anthropometric indexes of abdominal visceral adipose tissue accumulation and related cardiovascular risk in men and women. *Am J Cardiol* 1994;73:460–8

23. Pietrobelli A, Formica C, Wang Z, Heymsfield SB. Dual-energy X-ray absorptiometry body composition model: review of physical concepts. *Am J Physiol* 1996;271:E941–51

24. Sjostrom L, Kvist H, Cederblad A, Tylen U. Determination of total adipose tissue and body fat in women by computer tomography, 40K, and tritium. *Am J Physiol* 1986;250:E736–45

25. Gray DS, Fujioka S, Collette PM, *et al*. Magnetic-resonance imaging used for determining fat distribution in obesity and diabetes. *Am J Clin Nutr* 1991;54:623–7

26. Haarbo J, Marslew U, Gotfredsen A, Christiansen C. Postmenopausal hormone replacement therapy prevents central distribution of body fat after menopause. *Metabolism* 1991;40:1323–6

27. Gambacciani M, Ciaponi M, Cappagli B, *et al*. Body weight, body fat distribution, and hormonal replacement therapy in early postmenopausal women. *J Clin Enodcrinol Metab* 1997;82:414–17

28. Espeland MA, Stefanick ML, Kritz-Silverstein D, *et al*. Effect of postmenopausal hormone therapy on body weight and waist and hip girths. *J Clin Endocrinol Metab* 1997;82: 1549–56

29. Gambacciani M, Ciaponi M, Cappagli B, De Simone L, Orlandi R, Genazzani AR. Prospective evaluation of body weight and

body fat distribution in early postmenopausal women with and without hormonal replacement therapy. *Maturitas* 2001;39:125–32

30. Sites CK, Brochu M, Tchernof A, Poehlman ET. Relationship between hormone replacement therapy use with body fat distribution and insulin sensitivity in obese postmenopausal women. *Metabolism* 2001;50:835–40

31. Walker RJ, Lewis-Barned NJ, Sutherland WH, *et al*. The effects of sequential combined oral 17beta-estradiol norethisterone acetate on insulin sensitivity and body composition in healthy postmenopausal women: a randomized single blind placebo-controlled study. *Menopause* 2001;8:27–32

32. Anderson EJ, Lavoie HB, Strauss CC, Hubbard JL, Sharpless JL, Hall JE. Body composition and energy balance: lack of effect of short-term hormone replacement in postmenopausal women. *Metabolism* 2001;50:265–9

33. Davis SR, Walker KZ, Strauss BJ. Effects of estradiol with and without testosterone on body composition and relationship with lipids in postmenopausal women. *Menopause* 2000; 7:395–401

34. Dobs AS, Nguyen T, Pace C, Roberts CP. Differential effects of oral estrogen versus oral estrogen–androgen replacement therapy on body composition in postmenopausal women. *J Clin Endocrinol Metab* 2002;87:1509–16

Studying the complexity of the menopause transition from an epidemiological perspective

5

M. F. Sowers

Introduction

From a clinical and epidemiological point of view, the menopause is an important life process, making a potential contribution to the physiological and psychological health of women and the social environments in which those women function. However, the menopausal transition period, extending from a time of active reproductive capacity with well-formulated hormone profiles through reproductive senescence and the relative absence of an ovarian contribution to a woman's hormone profile, has been less well studied than any other period of the lifespan except extreme old age.

This is an important period to understand. During this period, changes in the neuro-endocrine system and ovary may be included in a biological system in which aging is occurring in a more compressed time span or under a different control mechanism than in other organs such as the liver, heart or kidneys. This system is influenced by both social and biological factors; therefore, ovarian senescence provides a unique model for the study of aging-related processes. Second, specific characteristics of this transitional period (including duration, intensity and age at menopause) may influence short-term health and quality-of-life status and subsequent life expectancy.

There is limited evidence about stages of the menopause transition and the implications of those transition stages for short-term health or health status one to two decades following the transition. The collaboration of the endocrinologist, gynecologist and epidemiologist is required to develop and solidify a body of evidence to justify both prevention and intervention activities. Nonetheless, some of the paucity of information about the menopause is related to the complexity of studying the menopause in populations of women. In this presentation, we consider some of those challenges including the generation of case definitions for menopause, the role of confounding and effect modification, as well as the representativeness of study findings.

Case definitions

One of the first requirements for any clinical or epidemiological condition is a case definition. With case definitions, the clinician can consider appropriate intervention strategies. With a case definition, investigators can ascertain prevalence (the proportion of women in pre-, peri-, or postmenopause at a given time) or incidence (the proportion of women who become pre-, peri-, or postmenopausal when they were not in that state previously). To relate elements of the menopausal transition to health status, a case definition is a prerequisite. However, the menopause transition is plagued by case definitions that are difficult to reproduce and of unknown sensitivity and specificity with respect to both short-term and long-term sequelae. Case definitions are often discordant, particularly when comparing definitions based on menstrual cycle bleeding characteristics, symptoms and hormone concentrations.

The most frequently used case definition of the menopause was developed by a World Health Organization (WHO) consensus panel[1]. The menopause was defined as the permanent cessation of menstruation resulting from loss of ovarian follicular activity. This attribution is made in retrospect following 12 months of amenorrhea not associated with other factors such as pregnancy, lactation or known medical intervention. The perimenopause (or climacteric) was defined to include the period prior to the menopause as well as the first year following the menopause. The postmenopause was defined as the period after the menopause and begins following 12 months of spontaneous amenorrhea (Figure 1).

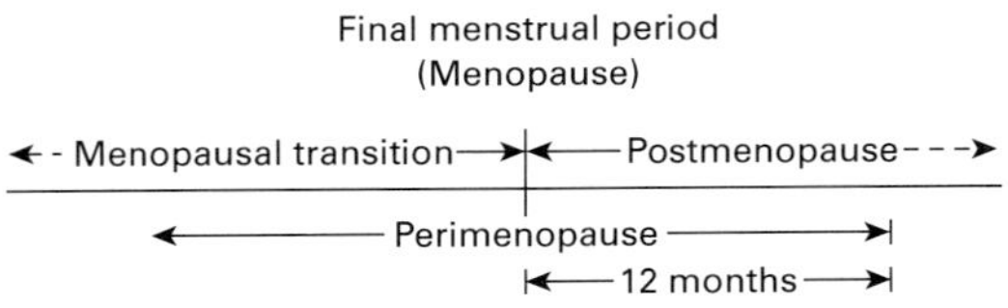

Stages of the menopause

An important issue with respect to case definitions of the menopause has been to identify 'stages' of the menopause transition leading to the last menstrual period (LMP) and the postmenopause. In studies of puberty, it has been useful to have a schema that describes the stages of development to characterize what is considered a normal or expected fulfilment in a transitional period. Similar approaches have been proposed for application to the menopause. Stages of the menopause are of interest if:

(1) Stage characteristics are predictive of subsequent stages;

(2) Stage characteristics facilitate clinical evaluation;

(3) Stage characteristics such as duration and age of onset are markers for subsequent health or disease status;

(4) Stage characteristics interact with lifestyle or genetic characteristics to create a dynamic environment that influences subsequent health or disease;

(5) Stage characteristics become an information tool with which to educate women at midlife;

Figure 1 Relationship between different time periods surrounding the menopause, employing World Health Organization definitions. Reproduced with permission

(6) Stages set a biological timeline in which prevention or intervention practices are optimally implemented.

The need for addressing case definitions was reflected in a July 2001 workshop held in Park City, Utah to propose a staging system for reproductive aging and to clarify nomenclature for the process of reproductive aging. The workshop was co-sponsored by the American Society for Reproductive Medicine, the National Institutes on Aging, the National Institute of Child Health and Human Development and the North American Menopause Society. As reproductive aging is a process and not an event, the purpose of a staging system was to identify when a given woman has entered the period of reproductive aging and when she passed through key stages of the reproductive aging process. A critical aspect of the workshop's recommendations was the development of an initial consensus regarding the specific menstrual and hormonal changes that characterize the transition from one stage to the next. The Stages of Reproductive Aging Workshop (STRAW) proposed that reproductive life could be characterized by stages during the reproductive years and during the transition years[2].

In earlier work, some investigators had described three stages of the menopausal transition, while others have described five stages[3,4]. For example, in the proposed first phase of menopause transition, there is an increase in follicle stimulating hormone (FSH) secretion, without a concomitant increase in the luteinizing hormone (LH) level[4]. Research has indicated a reduction in the secretion of inhibin and follistatin, peptides that inhibit

Table 1 Hormonal changes in the perimenopause according to the three proposed stages of menopausal transition (see text)

Hormone	Phase I	Phase II	Phase III
Estrogen	high relative to progesterone	high relative to progesterone	< 20 pg/ml
Progesterone	dropping	dropping	unmeasurable
FSH	slight increase	increasing levels	> 50 pg/ml
LH	non-responsive to FSH	non-responsive to FSH	elevated
FSH : LH ratio			> 1.0
Ovulatory cycles	premature ovulation	erratic	none

FSH, follicle stimulating hormone; LH, luteinizing hormone

the release of FSH from the pituitary gland in a closed feedback system with FSH. There is an increasing likelihood of premature ovulation, more frequent decrease of progesterone production with luteal insufficiency[4–6], hyperestrogenism in ovulatory cycles[7,8] and an excess of estrogen relative to progesterone. Characteristics of the perimenopause include a decline in the number of ovarian follicles to a depleted state in the postmenopause and a decrease in the proportion of ovulatory cycles[9].

The second proposed phase of the menopausal transition is characterized by an even greater instability in estrogen levels and an increasing probability of anovulatory cycles[10], with an apparent failure to mount an LH surge in response to an estrogen stimulus[5]. Abnormalities of the gonadotropin releasing hormone (GnRH) pulse generator affecting follicular[9] and luteal phases[11] as well as premature pulsatile LH secretion have been reported. Gonadal hormone levels are erratic with hyperestrogenism relative to progesterone[12] and altered presentation of menstrual cycle lengths and bleeding patterns[10,13–15]. This may include an increased frequency of dysfunctional uterine bleeding attributable to anovulation.

In the final proposed phase of the menopausal transition, the ovarian follicles no longer respond to FSH and LH. Plasma estradiol concentrations drop below 20 pg/ml and progesterone concentrations are non-measurable. Menstrual bleeding ceases. FSH and LH levels are consistently elevated, remaining so for an extended period of time[12,16–18] (Table 1).

Currently, these stages are on a poorly defined continuum that may not be discernible as discrete phases with a well-defined onset or specific points in time in every woman. Thus, the duration and progression of these phases toward the menopause, and the sources of variation in their presentation, duration and progression within groups of women, are areas of active epidemiological investigation.

It is necessary that staging definitions encompass patterns of menstrual bleeding, symptomatology or alterations in functioning, since these are the characteristics to which the woman and her clinical health-care provider are likely to respond. To achieve concordance of these domains with respect to a classification of the stages of the menopausal transition will require extensive epidemiological data and appropriate quantitative techniques. Such data must include longitudinal measures of symptoms and menstrual bleeding, as well as appropriate hormone and health measures; clinical trials will not provide the requisite information.

Measurement validity in definitions

Case definitions are based on menstrual bleeding, symptoms, hormone concentrations or health status. Each choice for a case definition has its own characteristics that limit or enhance its utilization. Symptoms and change in bleeding characteristics can be based on participant or client response and are identifiable by interview. There are several challenges to the fidelity of these self-reports. One assumption is that all respondents will have equal understanding of the nature of the events that the respondent is being asked to recall. However, there have been a number of reports that have suggested that cultural/ethnic groups may describe symptoms differently or their vocabulary/language does not encompass parallel symptom constructs. For example, it has been argued that Japanese women are less likely to have menopausal symptoms, but one reason that they may report fewer symptoms is that the Japanese have a vocabulary surrounding menopause symptoms that is not paralleled by the English vocabulary.

If the definition is based on hormone concentrations, then other aspects of measurement error, apart from recall and vocabulary, become important. In the measurement of hormone concentrations related to the menopausal transition, there will be greater laboratory variability. Normal curves titrated to the usual clinical range of hormones such as estradiol are likely to be inadequate to encompass both the lowest and the highest values that are found in the menopause transition. Furthermore, for adequate characterization of hormone concentrations, epidemiological and clinical studies must account for the cyclic variations in hormone concentrations including diurnal variation, menstrual cycle variation and minute-to-minute cycling. Thus, in the Study of Women's Health Across the Nation (SWAN), the date and time of phlebotomy are recorded and particular emphasis is placed on collecting samples before 10:00 h in fasted participants who are within days 2–5 of initiation of menstrual bleeding[19]. Figure 2 shows the variation that can occur in FSH concentrations according to when blood samples are drawn in the 1–7 day window of the early follicular phase of the menstrual cycle in pre- and early perimenopausal women when concentrations should be least variable (J.F. Randolph, M.F. Sowers, E.B. Gold, and associates, unpublished data).

Further, in SWAN, approximately one-quarter of the 3300 enrollees are collecting urine samples on a daily basis during one menstrual cycle for use with urinary hormone

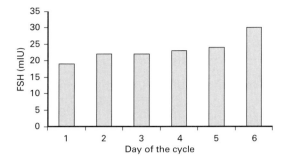

Figure 2 Mean follicle stimulating hormone (FSH) concentrations according to day of phlebotomy in the early follicular phase of the menstrual cycle. Adapted from SWAN data

assays. The goal of this activity is to clarify the nature of variation in cycling characteristics and the 'communication' of cycles with respect to ovulation and menstrual bleeding, and to determine those changes that aggregate together in what could be considered a 'stage' in the transitional process.

Defining when the menopause transition commences

Early age at menopause has been suggested as a biological marker of the general health status and aging of the individual woman[20,21]. While the WHO definition of the menopause considers when the 'perimenopause' ends, there are no well-accepted measures of when the 'perimenopause' commences. If earlier age at menopause is an important biological marker, one could hypothesize that the age of initiation of the perimenopause could also be an important health marker. Added to that, the duration and intensity of the perimenopause may stand as important elements of the woman's health, particularly when one considers that a perimenopausal period of 10 years would represent one-fifth of the life experience of the woman to that point.

Defining the onset of the perimenopausal period is particularly problematic for epidemiological studies. Many studies, including

Table 2 The frequency (%) of early ovarian failure, by ethnic groups in the SWAN cohort, can generate cohort effects that are particularly problematic in defining 'natural history' in cross-sectional studies. Adapted from unpublished data by J. Luborsky, P. Meyer, M.F. Sowers, *et al.*

Age at natural menopause (years)	Caucasian	African-American	Hispanic	Chinese	Japanese	Total
30–40						
% in ethnic group	1.0	1.4	1.4	0.5	0.1	1.1
40–45						
% in ethnic group	2.9	3.7	4.1	2.2	0.8	3.1

SWAN and the Melbourne Women's Health Study, commence observation of the natural history of the menopause at 42 and 45 years, respectively. To establish the average age at onset for the perimenopause requires that data collection be initiated prior to the perimenopause, so that a solid baseline is established from which greater variation can be measured. Although health-care providers have attempted to use the FSH concentration as the indicator of the onset of the perimenopause, FSH concentrations probably begin to change prior to age 42–45 years. However, the FSH concentrations have not been used to define the onset of the perimenopausal period because of the well-recognized and substantial variations in concentrations due to minute-to-minute, daily and monthly cyclicity. Currently, FSH concentrations have insufficient sensitivity and specificity to be used as an appropriate classification tool for the onset of the perimenopausal period in individual women (J.F. Randolph, M.F. Sowers, E.B. Gold, and colleagues, unpublished data).

Study designs

A requirement for a case definition is that the investigator must generate a count of both the affected and the unaffected women with respect to menopause. This has major implications for the sampling frame that will be used in characterizing the menopause transition. It is well recognized that studies that arise from clinical samples, especially samples from specialty clinics, do not reflect the experience of the population at large. This non-representativeness is particularly problematic in studies of developmental processes such as menopause and puberty, which, unlike pathologies, will encompass the entire population. Women enrolled in clinical studies, especially those from tertiary care settings with specialty menopause clinics, are more likely to be ill with multiple conditions and/or reflect those with access to medical-care systems.

Many studies use a single time observation (a cross-sectional study design) under the assumption that age is a surrogate for time and that each chronological age panel within a study can be laid out side-by-side to provide a 'natural history' of the menopause. Specifically with menopause studies, this would assume that chronological age is equivalent to ovarian aging. This assumption can be particularly fallacious when the investigator is interested in examining the characteristics of different ages at menopause, identifying the beginning of perimenopause, defining stages of transition and the length of time in each stage of the transition. Further, this assumption is sensitive to cohort effects. As seen in Table 2, the frequency of early ovarian failure is remarkably different among African-American and Hispanic women compared with the Japanese (J. Luborsky, P. Meyer, M.F. Sowers, and co-workers, unpublished data). There are important race/ethnic cohorts for which chronological ages could represent very different menopause effects.

A study of natural menopause, conducted in a geographic area with a very high prevalence of total hysterectomy (between 25 and 40%), is likely to have a different age at menopause than that described in women from a geographic area in which there is limited medical intervention. Numerous factors can create 'cohort' effects. The generation of women who have extensively used oral contraceptives creates a cohort that may have a different perimenopause experience. Asian women with diets rich in genistein, diadzein and other isoflavones represent a different cohort. It is most important to select a sample that represents the experience of the largest number of women or to recognize when unique cohorts are being selected.

There is an increasing focus on menopause studies that use community-based samples or population-based samples to generate findings that are more representative of the total population of women. Community samples are from women who come from the community and are not linked specifically to the health-care system. These community samples are generated by identifying women through a variety of methods including lists of voters, clients of health management organizations or even driver's license holders. While these studies are certainly more representative of the entire population than are studies from clinical samples, they too are not fully representative of the population. The optimal study population to generate counts would be representative of an important population where the sampling fraction is known, so that findings could be extrapolated to that known population. A sampling fraction represents the percentage of the population represented by the women who are being evaluated for menopausal characteristics. The Michigan site of the SWAN used this approach by conducting a census of two communities, identifying all eligible women by age and menstrual status in those communities, and then sampling to ensure that a specified number of African-American women were incorporated into the data collection. Since sampling probabilities are known, the variation around the estimates of association can then be adjusted to reflect the proportion of African-Americans in the total population.

It is particularly important that studies of the menopausal transition include sampling frames that are rich in diverse populations of women. This diversity should include variation in race/ethnicity, socioeconomic and social structures and lifestyle practices. A highly positive attribute of the SWAN approach is that it includes five race/ethnic groups that have all been studied using the same protocol, so that differences that are identified can be attributed to the elements under study and not to differences in how measures were secured.

It is generally considered more rigorous to conduct studies that observe the event of interest (the menopause) rather than having women try to remember the events of the menopause. Thus, a prospective design would be less subject to recall bias than would a retrospective design such as a case–control study. However, even in a prospective study, it remains important to recruit populations of women that are representative of the population. As shown in Table 3, even with major efforts to recruit representative populations, persons who are less affluent and less educated, who engage in at-risk health practices such as smoking, or who are less healthy are not as likely to participate in research[19].

Confounding and effect modification

There is a major problem with confounding in studying menopause in a diverse population. As an example, confounding occurs when the association between race/ethnicity and the menopause status is biased (misstated) by a third factor that is associated with both race/ethnicity and the measures of menopause status. This third factor distorts the association if the investigator fails to adjust for it in either the study design or the statistical analysis.

A research question in SWAN is determining whether there is an association between race/ethnicity and estradiol and FSH hormone levels. In addressing this question, body mass

Table 3 The longitudinal SWAN cohort percentage participation among cohort-eligible Caucasian women according to sociodemographic and lifestyle characteristics. Adapted from reference 19

Subject characteristic	% of Caucasians participating in cohort
Education	
less than high school	25.0*
high school degree	31.8*
some college	51.4*
college degree	53.5*
post-college	61.1*
Smoking	
never smoked	51.4*
past smoking	51.6*
current smoking	39.2*
Difficulty in paying for basics	
very hard	40.0*
somewhat hard	45.1*
not hard at all	51.5*
Self-reported health status	
excellent	51.8
very good	49.4
good	45.9
fair	45.2
poor	40.9*
Menopause status	
premenopausal	48.4
early perimenopausal	49.4

*95% confidence intervals indicate a significant difference in participation between all levels of education, smoking behavior and ability to pay for basics. There is a significant difference in participation between those who consider themselves as poor in health compared to all others

index (BMI) is a confounder. There is an association between the hormone concentrations and ethnicity, with Chinese women having lower estradiol and FSH concentrations than Caucasian women of the same chronological age. Simultaneously, there is also an association of ethnicity with BMI. The same Chinese women who have different hormone profiles also have a significantly different BMI.

Typically, one could statistically adjust for the confounding effect by body size. However, accepted statistical approaches are sometimes difficult to apply in epidemiological studies of the menopause. As shown in Figure 3 using SWAN data, there is a limited overlap of the BMI among women of the five race/ethnic groups. In the SWAN cohort, BMI ranges from $15 \, kg/m^2$ to more than $50 \, kg/m^2$. Less than 10% of African-American and Hispanic women are in the lowest BMI quartile, while more than 50% of the Chinese and Japanese women are in the lowest quartile. In contrast, more than 40% of African-American women are found in the highest quartile of BMI distribution, yet less than 5% of Chinese and Japanese women are in the highest BMI quartile.

This example of confounding of body size and race/ethnicity means that alternatives should be considered. These include:

(1) Changing the question from 'Is there a race/ethnicity association with menopause-related hormones, after adjusting for BMI?' to 'Is there a BMI association with menopause-related hormone concentrations *within* the race/ethnic groups?'

(2) Changing the question from 'Is there a race/ethnicity association with menopause-related hormones, after adjusting for BMI?' to 'Is there a race/ethnicity association with menopause-related hormone concentrations within the second BMI stratum?' The reason for this is that it would be useful to be able to ask the question of interest in the area of the distribution where there are a reasonable number of data points to use statistical adjustment.

(3) Considering statistical approaches such as spline regression that allow comparisons without forcing comparisons that are not supportable by the data distribution.

(4) Beginning to look for effect modification. When a third variable, such as BMI, modifies the way race/ethnicity interacts with respect to menopause, the response is called effect modification. This would suggest that Chinese women with a BMI of $24.0 \, kg/m^2$ have a different hormone profile from that of Hispanic women with a BMI of $24.0 \, kg/m^2$. In the case of effect modification, the influence of BMI on hormone concentrations should

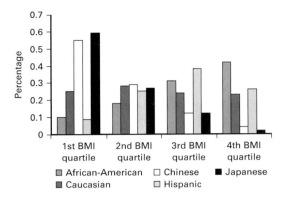

Figure 3 The confounding of body mass index (BMI) with ethnicity when trying to examine the association of either ethnicity or body size with menopause characteristics. Adapted from SWAN data

not be eliminated; rather its interaction with race/ethnicity should be explicitly considered.

In summary, the menopausal transition offers unique opportunities to consider health and aging. The transition is a model to consider both the intrinsic metabolic processes and the extrinsic factors. Nevertheless, ironically, the menopausal transition is a poorly characterized developmental stage with a potential to help understand aging processes that has barely been tapped. There are three constructs integral to the menopause transition itself that may reflect a matrix of physiological and sociological processes that both influence the immediate experience of the transition at midlife and may have long-term consequences for a woman, including her life expectancy. The three constructs include duration of the transition; age at menopause; and a marker of the intensity of the experience, observed as symptoms, shifts in hormone concentrations and ovarian function. The duration, intensity and placement on a chronological age scale can potentially have an immediate impact; however, even more intriguing is its potential to affect the 'programming' for total life expectancy for women. These complex dynamics are better studied in observational rather than experimental settings. However, the complex dynamics also pose challenges that must be addressed. Understanding these constructs will provide the evidence needed to address the contribution of the menopause transition to the health status of women.

Acknowledgements

SWAN was funded by the National Institute on Aging, the National Institute of Nursing Research and the Office of Research on Women's Health of the National Institutes of Health. Supplemental funding from the National Institute of Mental Health, the National Institute of Child Health and Human Development, the National Center on Complementary and Alternative Medicine, the Office of Minority Health, and the Office of AIDS Research is also gratefully acknowledged.

Clinical Centers: University of Michigan, Ann Arbor, MI (U01 NR04061, MaryFran Sowers, PI); Massachusetts General Hospital, Boston, MA (U01 AG12531, Robert Neer/Joel Finkelstein, PI); Rush University, Rush-Presbyterian-St. Luke's Medical Center, Chicago, IL (U01 AG12505, Lynda Powell, PI); University of California/Kaiser, Davis, CA (U01 AG12554, Ellen Gold, PI); University of California, Los Angeles, CA (U01 AG12539, Gail Greendale, PI); University of Medicine and Dentistry–New Jersey Medical School, Newark, NJ (U01 AG12535, Gerson Weiss, PI); and the University of Pittsburgh, Pittsburgh, PA (U01 AG12546, Karen Matthews, PI).

Laboratory: University of Michigan, Ann Arbor, MI (U01 AG12495, Daniel McConnell, PI) and Medical Research Laboratories (MRL), Highland Heights, KY (subcontract of U01 AG12553, Evan Stein, Director).

Co-ordinating Center: University of Pittsburgh, Kim Sutton-Tyrell, PI.

Project Officers: Taylor Harden, Carole Hudgings, Marcia Ory, Sherry Sherman.

Steering Committee Chair: Jennifer L. Kelsey.

This manuscript was reviewed by the Publications and Presentations Committee of SWAN and has its endorsement.

We thank the study staff at each site and all of the women who participated in SWAN.

References

1. World Health Organization. Report of a WHO Scientific Group. *Research on the Menopause*. WHO Technical Report Series 670. Geneva: WHO, 1981
2. Soules MR, Sherman S, Parrott E, *et al*. Executive summary: Stages of Reproductive Aging Workshop (STRAW). *Climacteric* 2001;4: 267–72
3. Sowers MF, La Pietra M. Menopause: its epidemiology and potential association with chronic diseases. *Epidemiol Rev* 1995;17: 287–302
4. Prior JC. Perimenopause: the complex endocrinology of the menopausal transition. *Endocr Rev* 1998;19:397–498
5. Metcalf MG, Donald RA, Livesey, JH. Pituitary–ovarian function before, during and after the menopause: a longitudinal study. *Clin Endocrinol* 1982;17:489–94
6. van Look PF, Lothian H, Hunter WM, Michie EA, Baird DT. Hypothalamic–pituitary–ovarian function in perimenopausal women. *Clin Endocrinol* 1977;7:13–31
7. Reyes FI, Winter JSD, Faiman C. Pituitary–ovarian relationships preceding the menopause. *Am J Obstet Gynecol* 1977;129:557–64
8. Santoro N, Brown JR, Adel T, Skurnick JH. Characterization of reproductive hormonal dynamics in the perimenopause. *J Clin Endocrinol Metab* 1996;81:1495–501
9. Shideler SE, DeVane GW, Kaira PS, Benirschke K, Lasley BL. Ovarian–pituitary hormone interactions during the perimenopause. *Maturitas* 1989;11:331–9
10. Klein NA, Battaglia DE, Miller PB, Branigan EF, Giudice LC, Soules MR. Ovarian follicular development and the follicular fluid hormones and growth factors in normal women of advanced reproductive age. *J Clin Endocrinol Metab* 1996;81:1946–51
11. Metcalf MG. Incidence of ovulatory cycles in women approaching the menopause. *J Biosoc Sci* 1979;11:39–48
12. Reame NE, Kelch RP, Beitins IZ, Zawacki CM, Padmanabhan V. Age effects of FSH and pulsatile LH secretion across the menstrual cycles of premenopausal women. *J Clin Endocrinol Metab* 1996;81:1512–18
13. Vagenakis AG. Endocrine aspects of menopause. *Clin Rheumatol* 1989;8:48–51
14. Treloar AE, Boynton RE, Behn BG, Brown BW. Variation of the human menstrual cycle through reproductive life. *Int J Fertil* 1967;12: 77–127
15. Vollman RF. *The Menstrual Cycle. Major Problems in Obstetrics and Gynecology*, vol 7. Philadelphia: WB Saunders, 1977
16. Rutherford AM. The menopause. *NZ Med J* 1978;87:251–3
17. Chakravarti S, Collins WP, Forecast JD, Newton JR, Oram DH, Studd JWW. Hormonal profiles after the menopause. *Br Med J* 1976;2: 784–7
18. Scaglia H, Medina M, Pinto-Ferreira AL, Vazques G, Gual C, Perez-Palacios G. Pituitary LH and FSH secretion and responsiveness in women of old age. *Acta Endocrinol* 1976;81: 673–9
19. Sowers MF, Crawford S, Sternfeld B, *et al*. Design, survey sampling and recruitment methods of SWAN: a multi-center, multi-ethnic, community-based cohort study of women and the menopausal transition. In Wren J, Lobo RA, Kelsey J, Marcus R, eds. *Menopause: Biology and Pathobiology*. San Diego: Academic Press, 2000
20. Snowdon DA, Kane RL, Beeson WL, *et al*. Is early natural menopause a biologic marker of health and aging? *Am J Public Health* 1989;79: 709–14
21. Cooper GS, Sandler DP. Age at natural menopause and mortality. *Ann Epidemiol* 1998; 9:229–35

Midlife sexuality

6

A. Altman

While research into female sexuality is still in its early stages, it has become clear that perimenopausal women do not present a common clinical picture of how this transition impacts their sexual lives. While many will notice little change, some may actually notice an improvement, and others will complain of diminished sexual function, often for the first time in their lives. The ramifications of erratic ovarian function and fluctuating hormone levels that define the perimenopause, and the more definite decline that follows the menopause, can upset even the smoothest sexual continuum into midlife. Add to this scenario alterations in anatomical structure, neurological function, vascular responsiveness and psychosocial function that accompany the normal aging process, as well as relationship dynamics and each individual's foundation of sexual beliefs, expectations and prior sexual experiences, and the resulting impact on midlife sexuality can be dramatic. Unfortunately, many women will not connect what is happening hormonally with what is happening sexually, and will not, therefore, seek the knowledge and treatment that could help. These changes present a unique opportunity for the clinician to ask the appropriate questions, bring the problem out into the open, and then offer counselling and guidance. This requires the ability to communicate comfortably with patients along with an understanding of the physiology of the human sexual response, the normal effects of aging on sexuality, relationship dynamics and the health-care provider's own limitations. These distinctions, and the treatment options available to the clinician to help maintain or restore sexual function, are the primary focus of this chapter.

Midlife

The concept of midlife must be redefined within the perspective of our ever-changing life expectancy. Women today actually experience two midlives: one reproductive, the other chronological, and the two do not necessarily coincide. In the past, with a life expectancy of 50–60 years, menopause generally appeared near the end of a woman's life, and midlife, chronologically, coincided with the reproductive changes in ovarian function beginning in the mid-thirties.

At the dawn of the third millennium, life expectancy has increased to the 80s and chronological midlife has come to be redefined as the fifties and sixties, while reproductive midlife remains unchanged. For women and their health-care providers, this discrepancy between a woman's reproductive midlife and her chronological midlife presents basic problems. It is difficult for women in their thirties to think of themselves as entering midlife, even though endocrine changes begin at that age, initiating the process of decline in reproductive function. Also, *when* midlife occurs will affect the kind of sexual changes that are experienced. The older midlife woman will tend to have more physiological and anatomical problems than the younger midlife woman, in whom psychosocial problems might predominate. Today, women and men expect sexual interest and function to continue for decades beyond the point where women lose their natural reproductive capabilities. Fortunately, the clinician can do much to help patients in reproductive midlife maintain sexual function well into and beyond chronological midlife.

Midlife sexuality

If midlife represents a variable state, so does midlife sexuality. While the host of hormonal and other changes that begin prior to the peri-menopausal transition and continue beyond the menopause affect sexuality, the desire for an active sex life remains important throughout midlife, as has been detailed in several recent surveys.

Dennerstein and co-workers surveyed 1879 women, aged 45–55 years (most of whom had partners) to identify changes in sexual interest over the previous year[1]. Of the respondents, 62% noted no change, 31% reported a decline in interest and 7% indicated an increase in interest. Of this last group, most had new partners.

A 1999 Modern Maturity Survey (AARP) asked responders aged 45 and older if they were more or equally satisfied with their current sex life, when compared with their past levels of sexual activity[2]. Of the males, 56% were more or equally satisfied, as were 51% of the females. When asked if individuals considered themselves 'a better lover now than in the past', 54.3% of the men and 37.6% of the women responded affirmatively.

The AARP survey also revealed that 70% of males and females with partners had intercourse one or two times a week. Of those without regular partners, 6% of males had intercourse one or two times a week; women had considerably less. Interestingly, females 45–59 years of age were more likely than males to approve sex outside marriage, oral sex, masturbation and sex as a normal part of aging. Age became a factor when the participants were asked, 'What would improve your sex life?' Men and women aged 45–59 cited less stress and more free time; men over 60, better health; women 60–74, better health for their partner; and women over 75 responded that just having a partner would improve their sex life.

Midlife can be a time of sexual freedom for many women; freedom from cycles, bleeding, sanitary pads and tampons, interruptions by small children and, of course, risk of unwanted pregnancy. These factors can enhance midlife sexuality, especially if sex was a positive experience earlier in the individual's life. However, some women see midlife as a loss of youth, femininity and childbearing capacity, leading to a negative impact on sexuality. Still others see midlife as a time when they can finally use these changes as a long-anticipated excuse to avoid sex that was never enjoyable for them before.

Sexual changes in midlife

Sexuality and sexual capacity evolve over a lifetime of development and change, based on personal experience, interest, cultural attitudes, interpersonal relationships, desires, behaviors, physiology and other factors.

As reproductive midlife approaches, this foundation of sexuality can be altered by anatomical, neurological, vascular, hormonal and neuropsychological changes. None of these categories, however, are mutually exclusive. They are all interrelated and it is unusual to find a change impacted by only one factor. For example, while vaginal dryness can be thought of as an anatomic change, it is directly related to the hormonal change of estrogen deficiency and to the resulting decrease in vaginal blood flow, a vascular change. This can result in painful sex, a neurological change, often followed by aversion to or avoidance of sex, a neuropsychological change.

Since a key factor for women is the impact of declining levels of sex hormones, this section will begin with a discussion of the physiological changes within this context and, later, address psychosocial and other issues.

Estrogen changes

Estrogen deficiency can occur gradually over time through the perimenopausal transition beginning in the mid- to late thirties and leading up to the last menstrual period, the menopause. A far more abrupt decline is seen with surgical menopause.

Urogenital atrophy

Estrogen sustains the structure and function of the cells of the vagina. Every woman who experiences estrogen deficiency for a prolonged period of time will develop some degree of vaginal and genital atrophy. Epithelial changes in the vagina occur first, within weeks to months of estrogen loss. This leads to a decrease in superficial cells, an increase in parabasal cells and a progressive loss of elasticity and the integrity of the epithelium. Along with this change comes an increase in vaginal pH, which promotes the growth of organisms and leads to more frequent vaginal infections[3]. Later changes, over years, affect the deeper structures such as the underlying vascular, muscular and connective tissues, leading to a decrease in vaginal blood flow, and both foreshortening and narrowing of the vagina. There is loss of blood vessels in the layers beneath the epithelium, responsible for the decrease in vaginal blood flow. This constellation of changes can lead to vaginal dryness, decreased or absent lubrication and, finally, dyspareunia. The bladder tissues also suffer from estrogen loss with mucosal changes that can lead to urinary frequency, urgency, nocturia, dysuria and incontinence. Clitoral changes are also noted, including a 50% decrease in perfusion and shrinkage of the structure[4]. Neurological changes include decreased touch perception, a decline in vibratory sensation and slowing of nerve impulses, leading to a delay in reaction time[5].

Effect on sexual response

Such changes in the vaginal and clitoral tissues can have a profound effect on sexual response. Beginning with the perimenopausal transition, the decrease in genital blood flow will affect vasocongestion. Sexual arousal will be delayed or altered. More time and stimulation may be necessary to achieve lubrication, which may be significantly reduced or absent. The outer third of the vagina, including the labia and G-spot, demonstrate decreased or absent congestion, as does the clitoris. Vaginal expansion in length and transcervical width decreases. Elsewhere, there is a decreased incidence of skin flush, a lack of increase in breast and nipple size during stimulation, decreased tactile sensation, or worse, aversion to skin touch due to pain perception instead of pleasure in the clitoris, skin and nipples, and a general decrease in muscle tension[6].

Taken together, these changes can result in delayed arousal, delayed or absent orgasm or diminished peak of orgasm. Fewer uterine contractions occur with orgasm, and in older women, particularly those aged 70 and older, painful uterine contractions can be associated with orgasm, a result of vasoconstriction that produces ischemia[4].

Androgens, aging and sexual response in women

Androgens in women are produced by the ovaries and adrenals throughout life. In fact, the normal ovary produces twice as much androgen as estrogen, and all estrogen begins as androgen. Pituitary luteinizing hormone (LH) stimulates ovarian production of androstenedione and testosterone from cholesterol. Follicle stimulating hormone (FSH) stimulates the aromatase enzyme system to convert androgens into estrone and estradiol[7]. The adrenal glands produce what are often referred to as the pre-androgens or androgen precursors, androstenedione, dehydroepiandrosterone (DHEA) and DHEA sulfate (DHEAS). While the ovary produces a great deal of testosterone, the peripheral conversion of pre-androgens is responsible for 50–75% of circulating testosterone (Figure 1).

Once testosterone is produced in the ovary or peripherally, it can take one of two paths: aromatization to estradiol, or reduction to its active metabolite, dihydrotestosterone. In this manner, testosterone can ultimately affect both estrogen and androgen receptors. Testosterone can also be aromatized to estradiol in the brain, bone, fat, skin, vascular endothelium, smooth muscle, cardiac myocytes, placenta and testes. Testosterone is the primary precursor for estrogen biosynthesis. Since all estrogen comes from androgens, if there is not enough androgen, there will not be enough estrogen. It might also follow that aromatase inhibitors might have a

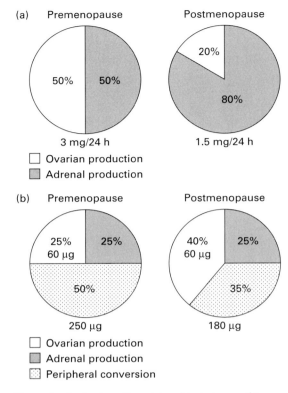

Figure 1 Androstenedione (a) and testosterone (b) production before and after the menopause. Adapted from references 8 and 9

use in the future for breast cancer therapy that may be more effective than tamoxifen.

Total testosterone declines with age in normal young women. Longcope and Johnston noted that androgen levels peak around age 25 and decline in the late thirties or early forties, much earlier in life than do estrogen levels[8]. The decline is most often manifested as an inconsistent or diminished sexual urge, although, during the reproductive cycle, many women experience a surge of testosterone mid-cycle designed to encourage sexual activity during ovulation. Still, when researchers compared women in their twenties with regular menses, with women in their forties with regular menses, they observed that the mid-cycle testosterone surge was either absent or significantly reduced in the older age group[10]. Table 1 shows these changes

in women's circulating androgen and estrogen levels.

Testosterone has other general effects, such as maintenance of muscle and bone, energy level, vascular endothelial function as well as vaginal blood flow and lubrication. More centrally, testosterone is involved with estrogen synthesis in the brain, and has pronounced psychological effects on well-being, mood, motivation and libido or desire. It is important to note that estrogens up-regulate androgen receptors; therefore, estrogen and androgens act synergistically and can improve some beneficial effects; for instance, combined estrogen–androgen therapy produces better effects on bone than does estrogen alone[12].

Increasingly, it is becoming apparent that testosterone may be important for libido, fantasy and drive for sexual activity[13]. Studies evaluating vaginal blood flow and vasocongestion of the clitoris and labia suggest that normal testosterone levels are necessary to allow arousal and orgasm to occur[14]. Some studies have demonstrated that testosterone increases sexual motivation, frequency of sexual activity and orgasm[15–17]. The family of androgens may be more important in its effects on sexual desire and libido, than are estrogens.

One school of thought hypothesizes that the improvement in sexual function that can result from administration of androgens is a manifestation of a central sex steroid effect on mood and sense of well-being. Others posit a specific role of androgens in enhancing the sexual response.

Androgen insufficiency

Androgen insufficiency is a theoretical syndrome that can affect women as a result of aging, hysterectomy, oophorectomy (producing a sudden 50% fall in levels within 24 h of surgery), chemotherapy or radiation therapy, gonadotropin releasing hormone (GnRH) agonist therapy, spironolactone use, steroid therapy suppressing adrenocorticotropic hormone (ACTH) secretion, adrenal insufficiency and enzyme defects. Other clinically relevant, acquired causes include exogenous

Table 1 Plasma steroid levels (mean ± SEM) in normal women. From reference 11

	Reproductive-aged women (n = 15)	Naturally menopausal women (n = 18)	Oophorectomized women (n = 8)
Estrone (pg/ml)	58 ± 16	49 ± 5	48 ± 6
Estradiol (pg/ml)	40 ± 3	20 ± 1	18 ± 4
Testosterone (ng/dl)	44 ± 2	30 ± 4	12 ± 2
Dihydrotestosterone (ng/ml)	30 ± 4	10 ± 2	< 5
Androstenedione (ng/dl)	166 ± 10	99 ± 13	64 ± 9
Dehydroepiandrosterone (ng/dl)	542 ± 21	197 ± 43	126 ± 36

Table 2 Binding of androgens to plasma proteins. From reference 20

Steroid	% unbound	% bound to albumin	% bound to SHBG
Dehydroepiandrosterone sulfate	5.0	95.0	—
Dehydroepiandrosterone	3.93	88.1	7.9
Androstenediol	1.73	19.4	78.8
Testosterone	1.36	30.4	66.0
Androstenedione	7.54	84.5	6.6

SHBG, sex hormone binding globulin

oral estrogens, such as oral contraceptives (OCs) and hormone replacement therapy (HRT), both of which increase sex hormone binding globulin (SHBG), resulting in reduced bioavailability of androgens (*and* estrogens). The condition is difficult to define with laboratory measurements of hormones, since immunoassays for testosterone generally lack the sensitivity to read the low levels found in women accurately. The condition is believed to be characterized by a loss of sexual desire, diminished sense of well-being, flat mood, loss of energy, decrease in assertiveness or confidence, and blunted motivation[18]. Over time, it can also result in decreased bone mass and muscle strength. Androgen insufficiency is believed to be linked to sexual dysfunction. Many women who report sexual dysfunction during the perimenopausal transition and later have actually been experiencing difficulty for years. Clinicians should be aware that the sexual effects of reduced androgen levels occur well before menopause and the onset of estrogen deprivation[19].

Generally, only 1–2% of the total amount of circulating testosterone is free or biologically available. Of the remainder, SHBG binds approximately 66%, albumin 30% and cortisol binding globulin 2% (see Table 2). Estrogens greatly affect the bioavailability of androgens, especially testosterone. Elevated levels of estrogen, such as those obtained from administration of exogenous oral estrogens, cause increased production of SHBG by the liver. SHBG preferentially binds testosterone, but also binds estrogen and some progesterone. Levels of SHBG are also increased by thyroxin. Importantly, they are decreased by testosterone, as well as by obesity, growth hormone, glucocorticoids and insulin resistance. For this reason, it is difficult accurately to assess levels of bioavailable testosterone. Indirectly, a likely diagnosis of androgen deficiency can be made when normal total testosterone levels accompany high levels of SHBG. This finding implies that levels of free testosterone and other androgens will be lower than normal because of elevated SHBG (see Diagnosis, p. 48).

The clinician treating peri- and postmenopausal women should be aware that supplementation with oral estrogen, especially without adding an androgen, can diminish bioavailable testosterone in two ways: first, by increasing SHBG; and second, by negative feedback reduction of LH, thereby reducing production of testosterone by the ovaries. While all oral estrogens such as in OCs and HRT will have this effect to some extent, conjugated equine estrogens (CEEs) can increase SHBG by up to 300%.

Androgens and the perimenopause

The perimenopausal transition results in a somewhat unique hormonal profile. The erratic function of the ovaries results in estrogen levels that can be normal, elevated or decreased at any given time. Ultimately, lower levels predominate which gradually cause a decrease in SHBG production and a resultant increase in bioavailable testosterone. In some women, if these levels are too high, it can lead to an increase in aggression, sexual tension and outbreaks of anger, often treated unsuccessfully with psychotropic therapy[21]. What is needed is oral estrogen supplementation to increase SHBG and diminish these levels. However, other women notice a pleasant increase in libido and desire for sexual activity or no change at all. More commonly, however, the perimenopause can herald the first signs of an androgen deficiency syndrome, beginning in the mid- to late thirties, due to the normal decrease in levels with aging, otherwise unaffected by reproductive senescence. When this is added to the multiple other midlife tensions, sexual desire and coital frequency can diminish to a point that both partners notice. It is in this last scenario that the addition of OC therapy to treat the erratic function of the ovaries, an important therapeutic modality for the overly symptomatic patient, can further diminish bioavailable testosterone and possibly add to the decline in sexual desire.

Common origins and important differences

While the discussion thus far has focused on female sexuality, it is useful to review the many similarities shared by both women and men in their sexual response, as this can have an impact on therapeutic options and results.

The physiology of sexual response with respect to neurovascular events leading to vasocongestion is quite similar in both sexes, which is not surprising since male and female genitalia originate from homologous structures. During early fetal development, the undifferentiated genital tubercle differentiates into either male or female genitalia. In the male, this structure develops into the glans penis, the shaft and the scrotum, while in the female, the clitoris, labia and the lower third of the vagina are formed. It follows, logically, that the same factors that cause erectile dysfunction in the male should cause problems with vasocongestion and, ultimately, arousal in the female. From there we can infer that modalities utilized to correct erectile dysfunction should also have an impact on sexual arousal dysfunction in women.

While physiological elements of the arousal phase are similar for men and women, important gender-specific differences exist in the motivational aspects of sexuality – the factors that drive desire. Leiblum has pointed out that males are, in general, high-desire individuals and are peripherally directed[22]. They are more urgent, more driven by fantasy, more goal-oriented, less distractible, and more focused on coitus and orgasm.

Females, however, are more centrally focused and more often motivated by desire for intimacy as opposed to a need for sexual release. They are more diffuse, more distractible and more receptive. Despite these broad conceptual differences, with the new equality in the bedroom, some women are becoming as goal-oriented as men, leading to some men feeling threatened because they are not 'running the show'. This leads to other role and relationship issues, which are important to sexual function and will be discussed later in this chapter.

One of the major factors that have an impact on female sexuality is the spectrum of midlife sexual changes in the male. Overall, men experience a decrease in testosterone production, penile sensitivity, libido, ejaculate and genital blood flow that can lead to diminished vasocongestion and alteration in achievement, maintenance and firmness of erection. These changes often lead to male performance anxiety, one of the most significant midlife sexual problems to have an impact on female midlife sexuality. When the male experiences performance anxiety, he will frequently withdraw from intimacy at all levels of the relationship for fear of stimulating his partner's desire for sexual activity he cannot provide. This withdrawal can have a profound impact on the relationship.

Libido or sexual desire

Decreased libido or sexual desire has increasingly become one of the more common complaints of women in the perimenopausal transition and in midlife in general. Sexual desire includes sexual appetite, drive and fantasy – basically what motivates the individual to seek sexual stimulation. While sexual arousal leading to orgasm is predominantly a physiological event dependent upon neurovascular responses to stimuli within the appropriate hormonal milieu, libido or sexual desire is more psychosocial and behavioral, affected by a multitude of factors that play a role in each individual woman's daily life and relationships. All roads lead to libido, and many roadblocks can detour even the best of intentions, including the impact of stress due to relationship issues, family pressures, job tensions and even the health-care needs of aging parents. Indeed, the hormonal milieu remains important here as well, but the desire for sexual intimacy can be diminished in spite of normal levels of testosterone and estrogen.

Many women see midlife as the opportunity for a more enjoyable sex life without monthly cycles and unexpected bleeding or the risk of pregnancy. They enjoy the freedom to take part in sexual encounters when they choose, not when their reproductive cycles dictate, and view a decline in sexual desire as a problem. Other women who engage in sexual activity because they feel obliged to do so, look forward to midlife as a source of relief from sexual demands. The clinician should note that absence of sexual activity is, in itself, not a problem. It should be viewed and treated as a problem only when a woman or her partner feels a problem has developed.

Many factors affect sexual drive and its expression in midlife and should be evaluated by the clinician whose patients present with decreased libido.

Partner availability

Women tend to live longer than men, resulting in a natural shortage of males aged 50 and older. At the same time, many men seek out younger partners, further affecting the male-drain and availability of partners for women in midlife and beyond. A welcomed change, noted recently, has been the increasing tendency for older women to seek out younger men. This is a fascinating change considering that, in many primitive societies, older men took younger women, giving their genes a higher chance of being passed to a subsequent generation via the more fertile females, and older women took younger, inexperienced men, allowing them to impart their wisdom and sexual experience.

Personal well-being

A woman's sense of personal well-being is of importance to sexual interest and activity. It has been shown that low perceived levels of both physical and emotional satisfaction and a sense of unhappiness correlate with low sexual desire, resistance to arousal and pain during sex[23]. Women who have experienced premenopausal physical or emotional problems, particularly disorders of sexual desire, sexual response and sexual behavior, tend to experience a worsening of these conditions after menopause[4].

Overall health and socioeconomic circumstances

Analysis of data from the National Health and Social Life Survey of 1749 women and 1410 men indicated that sexual dysfunction is highest in women with poor health, low income and a history of infrequent sexual interest. Also, it is more likely among women *and* men with poor physical and emotional health[23].

History

Desire is also influenced by a person's sexual knowledge and past experiences. Upbringing in an environment based on strict religious or moral codes that discouraged sexual feeling or release can have a long-lasting impact on sexual desire many years after the imprinting has occurred. Experience, especially the earliest, can sometimes set the tone for a lifetime of satisfaction or frustration, while a situation involving abuse can destroy any thought of sexuality, necessitating intense therapy to allow even a rudimentary realignment of a person's sexual being.

Performance anxiety

While far more is written about performance anxiety in men, it can also occur in women, usually because of a fear of pain or a fear of failure to be satisfied or to satisfy a partner. Recurrent dyspareunia can lead to introital spasm, which can lead to further pain, a potent diffuser of sexual desire. Erectile dysfunction in the male can lead to secondary performance anxiety in the female as she avoids sexual contact for fear of exposing her partner to potential failure on his part, or her perceived inadequacy to 'turn him on'.

Body image

While a small portion of the broadcast and print media has begun to change its long-held body image message, the vast majority still extol often unachievable appearances. Add to this television programs and movies that seek to convince the public that the people next door are having great sex and bed-rocking orgasms, the images midlife women have of themselves are bound to suffer from inadequacies. While these are issues that affect women (and increasingly men) of all ages, they become particularly problematic within the context of perimenopause and midlife sexuality. Incidental to the perimenopausal transition, the body's metabolic rate begins to slow and the same effort that years before was put into losing weight is now spent trying, often

unsuccessfully, to maintain it. Hormonal changes and the normal aging process also lead to negative effects on skin health, muscle tone and maintenance, and overall body conditioning. This scenario can weigh heavily on midlife sexuality. Women are often concerned that, without the ideal body, they will be neither desirable nor able to please their partner sexually – another kind of performance anxiety. 'We're not sexually active because I don't want him to see me naked'; 'We only have sex with the lights out or under the covers'; 'I'm never on top any more because I'm embarrassed by my sagging breasts and jiggling stomach'. This 'spectatoring', as described by Masters and Johnson[24], can limit a woman's ability to enjoy sex by causing her to be self-conscious and more concerned about how she looks during the act than how enjoyable it is. Body image can be totally independent of body weight. A woman who weighs 270 lb (120 kg) may have a healthy body image and a very active and enjoyable sex life, while one who weighs 135 lb (60 kg) and considers herself 'obese' has a very poor body image that may lead to an essentially non-existent sex life. The growth of body-image counselling is an understandable result of the scope of this problem.

Relationship issues

For women and their partners, especially in long-term relationships, midlife creates both opportunities and challenges that can affect sexual function. The sexual/marital equation implies that when there are sexual problems, they impact the marital relationship, and when there are marital problems, they impact the sexual relationship. It has also been said, 'When sex is good, it's 10% of a marriage; when it's bad, it's 90% of a marriage'. Issues of which the clinician should be aware include the following.

Attraction

Men and women change over the years, frequently at different rates, to the extent that what originally attracted them to each other may no longer be relevant. Often, when a couple first meet, they are attracted to each other because they are so different. Years later those very differences may put a strain on their relationship. Just as differences can diminish attraction, sameness can lead to a growing boredom from familiarity with one another, as well as with sexual habits that never vary and become routine and unstimulating. The couple become like siblings instead of lovers. They know each other so well that when he approaches her to initiate a sexual encounter, her thoughts wander to some of his annoying or distasteful habits, which diminishes any potential for stimulation. These thoughts have been termed 'anti-fantasies'.

Communication

Communication issues remain among the major problems encountered in relationships of any duration. Regardless of the couple's history of communication, sexual difficulties can often shut the door to the appropriate discussion about a sexual problem that both partners are aware of, yet neither wants to bring up. They avoid discussion out of shame or fear of emotional impact on the partner. Left unaddressed, the problem looms even larger and can spread beyond the confines of the bedroom where it originated. These secrets can destroy not only sexual desire, but also the very foundation of the relationship. Faking orgasm to avoid embarrassment or hasten the end of lovemaking, or pretending to be asleep to avoid sex altogether, are just two obvious examples. A long history of communication problems may already have had an impact on the sexual life of the midlife couple, stemming from an inability to guide each other in understanding what works for each partner to achieve sexual satisfaction.

Power struggles and lack of respect and trust

Power struggles are often played out in the bedroom, where one partner may withhold sexual activity to punish the other for some transgression. Especially in a relationship where a woman feels otherwise powerless to influence a decision or behavior, the only power she may have is in this arena. Loss of respect or trust over the years can also culminate in sexual inactivity.

Affairs

'Human beings *can* be monogamous, but make no mistake: it is unusual and difficult. Aspiring monogamists are going against some of the deepest-seated evolutionary inclinations with which biology has endowed most creatures, *Homo sapiens* included.' In their book, Barash and Lipton revealed that, with the use of DNA fingerprinting, even amongst the most monogamous of species, cheating on the mate is common for both sexes. Their thesis points out the profound difference between social monogamy and sexual monogamy; the former common and achievable, the latter highly unreliable and biologically weak[25].

Within this context, midlife is notorious for affairs of the mind, heart or body. Over and above any evolutionary imperative, they most often occur because of needs not being met in the relationship. In fact, some affairs allow the primary relationship to continue, where it might otherwise have ended, by fulfilling the unmet need and removing the strain on the relationship. More commonly, however, they destroy the primary relationship by robbing it of intimacy, trust and sharing, leading to its ultimate demise. The partner involved in the affair can frequently find it impossible to respond sexually to the spouse. This is one of the major causes of 'sexual dysfunction' in midlife that remains unspoken[26].

Medical issues affecting midlife sexuality

Arrival at chronological midlife can be greeted by medical issues that may affect sexuality in either the woman or her partner. These problems can act to diminish the physical ability to perform sexually, as with coronary artery disease or arthritis (the most prevalent cause of sexual inactivity in the USA), or affect arousal and orgasm capability, as with neurological disorders such as multiple sclerosis, parkinsonism or sequelae of diabetes[23]. Alcohol and substance abuse can have a disabling effect on performance by altering erectile capability in the male and arousal in the female. Psychiatric or emotional problems can impact sexual function because of the particular disorder or, just as commonly, because of the treatment of the problem. In addition, ovarian function plays a pivotal role in the serotonergic system. Sexual interest and motivation may decline on this basis. The central nervous system (CNS) stimulation necessary for arousal may be delayed. Women predisposed to mood disorders may experience psychological difficulties. Feelings of depressed or flat mood affect well-being and may lessen interest in sexual activity.

Pelvic injury

More reports are appearing in the literature concerning damage to the pudendal nerves associated with bicycle riding[6]. Narrow racing seats put pressure on the nerves and blood supply extending from the sacral area, beneath and forward to the clitoris or penis and can affect the ability to achieve arousal and orgasm. Attempts have been made to produce better seats that might avoid this kind of chronic injury. Another common cause of injury to the female genitalia is childbirth injuries leading to pelvic relaxation syndrome, or scarring of the perineum or introitus, causing persistent dyspareunia.

Medications

Both prescription and over-the-counter medications have the capability of altering desire, arousal and orgasm function. Any medication that alters blood flow (such as antihypertensives), affects the CNS (such as psychotropic therapies) or dries the skin or mucous membranes (such as antihistamines) is a candidate for disruption of normal sexual function. The medicine cabinet is one of the first places about which the clinician should enquire

(Table 3). As previously mentioned, both HRT and OC therapy can adversely affect levels of bioavailable androgens by increasing SHBG. Also, the potent progestin medroxyprogesterone acetate has been shown to decrease vaginal blood flow and has a history of being utilized to decrease libido in sex offenders[27].

One of the major classes of medication that impacts sexuality is the selective serotonin reuptake inhibitors (SSRIs), frequently used to treat depression in the perimenopausal woman. The risk/benefit ratio with use of these agents is based on individual need and response. When depression is severe, SSRIs may allow for increase in sexual activity by treating the underlying process. However, in many patients, female or male, this therapy can diminish sexual desire and alter or eliminate arousal and orgasm. (These properties have been utilized to treat premature ejaculation in men.) In a woman affected adversely by SSRI therapy, changing the agent may be helpful. The addition of bupropion to the ongoing therapy has been shown to improve sexual function (see Table 3).

Surgery

Surgery related to cancers of the breast or female genital tract can have a profound effect on sexuality in midlife, as can prostate surgery in men, both as a result of its effects on body image and function, as well as the psychological sequelae of the cancer diagnosis and prognosis on patient and partner alike. Many of these malignancies preclude the use of hormonal therapies, leading to even further problems involving genital function. Extensive counselling can be sex saving in these couples. Referral to an appropriate counsellor is vital. Of course, any postoperative recovery period or complication can impact sexuality in midlife.

Hysterectomy

Still one of the more common surgical procedures performed in women in the USA,

Table 3 Common medications that affect female sexuality. Adapted from reference 28

Desire disorder
Antipsychotics
  barbiturates
  benzodiazepines (e.g. Ativan®, Valium®, Xanax®)
  lithium
  psychoactive medications (e.g. Prolixin®, Thorazine®)
  fluoxetine (Prozac®)
  tricyclic antidepressants (e.g. Elavil®, Anafranil®)
Cardiovascular/antihypertensives
  antilipid medications (e.g. Atromid®, Lopid®)
  β-blockers (e.g. Inderal®)
  clonidine (Catapres®)
  digoxin
  spironolactone (Aldactone®)
Hormonal preparations
  danazol
  GnRH agonists (e.g. Lupron®, Synarel®)
Others
  histamine H_2-receptor blockers and anti-reflux agents
    (e.g. Tagamet®, Zantac®, Reglan®)
  indomethacin (Indocin®)
  ketoconazole (Nizoral®)
  phenytoin sodium (Dilantin®)

Arousal disorders
Anticholineregics (e.g. ProBanthine®)
Antihistamines (e.g. Seldane®, Benadryl®)
Antihypertensives (e.g. Clonidine®, Aldomet®)
Psychoactive medications
  benzodiazepines (e.g. Valium®, Ativan®)
  MAO inhibitors
  SSRIs (e.g. Prozac®, Zoloft®)
  tricyclic antidepressants (e.g. Elavil®, Anafranil®)
  alcohol

Orgasm disorders
Amphetamines and related appetite suppressants
Antipsychotics (e.g. Mellaril®, Thorazine®)
Benzodiazepines (e.g. Valium®, Xanax®, Ativan®)
Methyldopa (Aldomet®)
Naracotics (e.g. Methadone®)
SSRIs (e.g. Prozac®, Zoloft®)
Trazodone
Tricyclic antidepressants (e.g. Elavil®, Anafranil®)*

GnRH, gonadotropin releasing hormone; MAO, monoamine oxidase; SSRIs, selective serotonin reuptake inhibitors
*Also associated with painful orgasm

hysterectomy, with or without ovarian preservation, can have significant effects on hormonal, physiological and psychological function with respect to alterations in sexuality.

Avoidance of hysterectomy, unless all other therapeutic modalities have been unsuccessful, is the first step toward avoiding potential sexual problems. If unavoidable, and the indications are benign pathology, maintenance of adequate vaginal length is one important factor to allow successful and comfortable penetration postoperatively. This is usually more of a problem when removing the uterus through an abdominal incision, as opposed to vaginally. Two other important and somewhat controversial issues currently under debate are cervical and ovarian preservation.

In the process of female sexual arousal, the upper portion of the vagina expands and elevates cephalad with the uterus. This persists through orgasm and gradually returns to its neutral location with the resolution phase. A great deal of discussion has focused upon the possible role of the nerves and vascular structures that cross through the base of the broad ligaments at the vaginal apex. Does removal of the cervix and resulting disruption of the continuity of these neurovascular elements impact arousal and orgasm? Does penile 'bumping' of the cervix during intercourse add to sexual pleasure in some women? What are the risks of cervical stump cancer in women appropriately monitored with Pap smears? Is there a lower incidence of vaginal prolapse or enterocele formation with cervical preservation? There is some evidence to suggest that supracervical hysterectomy may avoid some of these sexual and structural problems[29], but data are sparse and emotions are high, especially when patients want options they have read about in the media or on-line. Many are now requesting that their ovaries be left *in situ* to allow for continued ovarian androgen production.

After hysterectomy, even when ovaries are left *in situ*, intraoperative ischemia, as well as ligation of the ovarian arteries, frequently result in diminished ovarian function. When ovaries are removed in the pre- or perimenopausal woman, the abrupt loss of hormones can cause major estrogen and androgen withdrawal symptoms that are far more severe than the symptoms associated with the gradual estrogen decline during a natural perimenopausal transition. It should be remembered that most vasomotor symptomatology occurs because of estrogen withdrawal, not simply because of low levels of estrogen, hence producing the more severe symptom complex. Also, one of the better defined clinical pictures seen in premenopausal women who have undergone hysterectomy and bilateral oophorectomy is that of androgen deficiency while on oral CEE therapy. Not only are the testosterone-producing ovaries gone, but also the small amounts of testosterone still being produced peripherally are bound up by elevated levels of SHBG from the CEE therapy; a double negative effect! Combined estrogen and androgen replacement in these women postoperatively should be considered.

Contrary to public perception, sexual function often improves with hysterectomy, although the relationship of the uterine corpus, itself, to sexual response remains under debate. Uterine contractions occur with orgasm in most women, although many are unaware of their presence. The seriousness of the pathology, along with the level of annoyance at bleeding, pain or pressure preoperatively, clearly affect satisfaction with sexual activity postoperatively. Rhodes and colleagues interviewed 1299 women prior to hysterectomy, and 1101 of these completed the study and provided information about sexual function[30]. The percentage that engaged in sexual relations increased significantly, from 70.5% before hysterectomy to 77.6% and 76.7% at 12 and 24 months, respectively, after surgery. The rate of frequent dyspareunia dropped significantly, from 18.6% before hysterectomy to 4.3% and 3.6% at 12 and 24 months, respectively (Figure 2). There remain, however, women who note a decrease or total absence of orgasm after hysterectomy. Preoperative counselling can help to prepare and assist the patient and partner by reviewing the risks of surgery, as well as the risks of not having the surgery, and potential sexual changes, better or worse, that might follow.

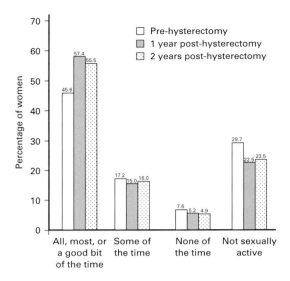

Figure 2 Frequency of orgasm before and after hysterectomy. From reference 30

Diagnosis of sexual dysfunction at midlife

For the gynecologist or other women's healthcare provider, the diagnosis of sexual dysfunction at midlife should begin with the use of the non-threatening question: 'Are you sexually active?' If the patient's answer is affirmative, the second question can be, 'Do you have any questions, problems or concerns about your sexual activity that you would like to discuss?' If, instead, the patient indicates that she is not sexually active, the next and most important question should be, 'Does that bother you or your partner?' There are two common reasons that these questions are not asked. First, the clinician may feel uncomfortable with such questions or with his or her level of knowledge of the subject. Second, there might be considerable time needed for discussion once the patient senses sincere interest and feels comfortable beginning a dialog with the provider. Especially in the managed care environment, it can be difficult to set aside the amount of time necessary for such a session. Often, it is useful, after initiating the discussion, to schedule a separate consultation at a later date so that more uninterrupted time can be spent, and also to allow the patient to gather all her thoughts on the topic she now knows is open for discussion. The presence of the partner can also be useful later, once the patient has covered her own concerns. Finally, within that consultation, a teaching session should occur, in which the clinician describes the normal sexual response as well as the physiological changes in sexuality that are common in midlife. Frequently, when patients realize so many of these changes are a normal part of the aging process and learn how to cope effectively with them, little or no therapy is needed. The point at which these physiological changes of aging become sexual dysfunction is best defined within the context of each individual relationship, based on the effect these changes have on the couple. The need for referral to a specialized counsellor, therapist, or sexologist should be made when more detailed consultation is necessary or when the clinician is simply unable to provide the service.

A detailed gynecological examination, as always, retains its importance. Careful assessment of the vulva, clitoris, introitus and vagina for atrophic changes, loss of elasticity, inflammation, scarring, infection or genital prolapse is paramount. Any tenderness to palpation, whether superficial or deep, must be evaluated. The pelvic structures, including the bladder, must be evaluated for pathology that might interfere with successful sexual activity; these include masses, endometriosis or urinary incontinence. Ultrasound imaging may be necessary as well.

For individuals with unresolved problems, laboratory tests can be performed to rule out other medical or endocrine problems. Assessment for levels of total and free testosterone, DHEAS and estrogens may be helpful, and some centers offer SHBG levels, which allow calculation of the free androgen index (FAI; the ratio of total testosterone to SHBG). As yet, there are no universal normal levels for androgens and each laboratory lists its own ranges. It should be noted that, in perimenopausal women, tests could be misleading because of the extremely erratic nature of ovarian estrogen/androgen production, and the relatively poor sensitivity of many commercially available androgen assays.

At this point, it may be useful to classify problems into one of four diagnostic categories created by the Consensus Panel of the American Foundation for Urologic Disease (AFUD)[31], based on the three-phase (desire, arousal, orgasm) model of female sexual response by Kaplan. These are often less useful for the clinician than for the research team.

(1) Sexual desire disorders

   (a) Hypoactive sexual desire disorder (HSDD); 'the persistent or recurrent deficiency (or absence) of sexual fantasies, and/or desire for, or receptivity to, sexual activity, which causes personal distress'

   (b) Sexual aversion disorder (SAD); 'the persistent or recurrent phobic aversion to and avoidance of sexual contact with a sexual partner, which causes personal distress'

(2) Female sexual arousal disorder (FSAD); 'the persistent or recurrent inability to attain or maintain sufficient sexual excitement, causing personal distress'

(3) Female orgasmic disorder; 'the persistent or recurrent difficulty, delay in, or absence of attaining orgasm following sufficient sexual stimulation and arousal, which causes personal distress'

(4) Sexual pain disorders

   (a) Dyspareunia; 'recurrent or persistent genital pain associated with sexual intercourse'

   (b) Vaginismus; 'recurrent or persistent involuntary spasm of the musculature of the outer third of the vagina that interferes with vaginal penetration, which causes personal distress'

   (c) Non-coital sexual pain disorder; 'recurrent or persistent genital pain induced by non-coital sexual stimulation'

The complaint of sexual dysfunction in both women and men can be a diagnostic window into other organ system function. Decreased blood flow to the genitalia can be a result of atherosclerotic plaque, which may be present elsewhere, impeding blood flow as well. Coronary or renal artery disease has been discovered secondary to erectile or arousal dysfunction. Diabetes can be involved with neurological problems first manifested as diminished sexual sensation or response.

Non-pharmacological treatment for sexual dysfunction at midlife

For those patients not satisfied with education alone, treatment can begin with any of a number of non-pharmacological initiatives. 'Use it or lose it' is a concept that is often discussed by providers of women's health care with their patients. While the phrase is principally intended to refer to the vagina and sexual activity, it can also apply to many other organ systems as well. The brain is a remarkably efficient organ. It directs blood flow to where it is needed. During the eating of a meal, blood flow is increased to the gastrointestinal tract; during exercise, to the musculoskeletal system; when body temperature is high, to the skin, etc. The same holds for the genitalia; blood flow increases during sexual activity. Hence, sexual activity begets better sexual function. In their early work, Masters and Johnson demonstrated that sexual activity maintains vaginal pH, po_2 and mucosal health and allows successful function to continue. In fact, the same beneficial effects can be achieved with sexual activity of any kind, partnered or unpartnered, including masturbation or basic sexual fantasy; sexual activity need not be defined solely as vaginal intercourse. Any sexual stimulation can have a similar effect on vaginal blood flow. Masturbation, either manually or through the use of vibrators or other sexual devices, need not include vaginal penetration to be beneficial, except with respect to keeping the introitus adequately patent. Similarly, sexual activity in males not only leads to an increase in blood flow, but also to increases in testosterone release if ejaculation occurs. In fact, lack of ejaculation can lead to decreased levels of testosterone. For both women and men in midlife, sex is good for continued sexual health.

Other non-pharmacological interventions include improved communication of sexual likes and dislikes; lifestyle changes including smoking cessation, adequate water intake and strength training; pelvic exercises with vaginal weights or biofeedback; more prolonged manual or oral stimulation; and altering the sexual routine to avoid sexual boredom.

Pharmacological treatment for female sexual dysfunction

In 1990, Sarrel conducted a short-term study to evaluate the effect of hormonal supplementation on sexual problems[32]. He reported that, of 93 women enrolled in the study, 68% reported problems with sex, specifically vaginal dryness of at least moderate degree (58%), dyspareunia (39%), decrease in clitoral sensitivity (36%), decrease in orgasmic frequency (29%), decrease in orgasm intensity (35%), decrease in sexual desire (77%) and intercourse once a month or less (50%). His findings demonstrated that, when estradiol levels dropped to below 50 pg/ml, women reported vaginal dryness, pain with penetration and a burning sensation. Symptoms decreased markedly when estradiol levels were above 50 pg/ml. Overall, oral estrogen therapy resulted in an improvement in clitoral sensitivity, and orgasm rates improved. The most dramatic response, however, was seen in the women who reported a lack of desire. After 3–6 months of treatment, 90% of these women had an increase in level of desire and increase in sexual activity.

Route of administration has also been evaluated. Prolonged therapy with oral estrogen ultimately increases SHBG, which can minimize not only bioavailable testosterone, but also bioavailable estrogen, potentially leading to diminishing benefits and even relapse of symptoms. The increase in SHBG appeared to be less significant in women who used non-oral delivery systems for estrogen replacement[33].

Effects of progestogens

Findings concerning the risk of endometrial hyperplasia resulting from the use of unopposed estrogen led to use of progestogens when an intact uterus was present. Prior to the micronization process, progesterone could not be used orally because of poor absorption and rapid breakdown. Synthetic progestins, some of which demonstrated very high potency, such as medroxyprogesterone acetate (MPA), were produced to allow for successful oral use. Progestational agents down-regulate the estrogen receptor, which is a desired result in the endometrium, but can be undesirable in the brain, heart, bone and genitalia. They generally have an overall negative effect in the CNS with respect to depression and mood, and have been shown to decrease sexual desire and diminish vaginal blood flow[34,35]. Newer options for progestational use in the USA for peri- and postmenopause now include micronized progesterone and the 19-nortestosterone derivatives norethindrone acetate and norgestimate. Micronized progesterone and norethindrone acetate have been extensively utilized outside the USA, where very little MPA is in use. Norethindrone acetate, the more androgenic progestin, has been shown to decrease SHBG and increase bone density, as would be expected from an androgen.

Sherwin compared the effects of estrogen alone or with MPA on psychological functioning and sexual behavior. The benefits of estrogen were diminished with MPA administration[34]. A comparison of estradiol alone or in combination with lynestrenol, a 19-norsteroid, revealed that women who used the combination therapy reported more negative mood symptoms than did the estrogen group[36]. In a single-arm, unblinded study, women who were intolerant of a CEE/MPA regimen were switched to CEE plus micronized progesterone and reported better vasomotor, somatic, psychological, cognitive and sexual functioning[35]. Progestogens seem to produce a wide range of patient responsiveness and tolerability, suggesting that patients who do not tolerate one regimen might be effectively switched to another and experience improvement. Newer studies in progress with more modern combinations of progestogens with estrogens will provide better insight into progestational effects on sexuality.

Effects of androgens

Although commonly thought of as male hormones, androgens are believed to play an important role in the physiological aspects of the female sexual response, so it is not surprising that they have been used to treat problems of sexual function and libido. Studies have demonstrated that testosterone in many forms results in increased sexual motivation, desire, fantasy and arousal, increased vaginal blood flow and lubrication, increased frequency of sexual activity and orgasm, increased pleasure and satisfaction, increased motivation and assertiveness, as well as improved mood and well-being[13,15–17]. Androgens are also associated with increase in lean body mass and bone formation, reduction in total body fat and improvement in estrogen-dependent vasodilatation. The potential risks of testosterone therapy include fluid retention, acne and hirsutism. Oral testosterone decreases triglycerides – especially the oral estrogen-induced increase in triglycerides – but also decreases high-density lipoprotein (HDL) cholesterol by up to 10%, although levels generally remain within the desirable range[12]. The major risks of hepatocellular damage and masculinization, including temporal balding, clitoromegaly and voice deepening, are very rarely seen with currently available doses. Some studies suggest the possibility of an association of endogenous androgens with decreased breast cancer risk, and exogenous testosterone has been associated with inhibition of estrogen-induced mammary epithelial proliferation and suppression of estrogen receptor expression in breast cells[37]. Recently, methyltestosterone has been shown to be a potent aromatase inhibitor and may find a future use in breast cancer prevention[38].

Studies looking at androgens and the effect of estrogen–androgen combinations on sexual function date to the 1950s. In a prospective double-blind placebo-controlled study published in 1950, Greenblatt and colleagues reported that estrogen/androgen improved libido and menopausal symptoms, and decreased breast tenderness, pelvic pain and nausea[15]. Five years later, Birnberg and Kurzrok presented a case series, noting that estrogen/androgen improved libido and mood, produced a better tonic effect, and were accompanied by either unchanged or lower blood pressure readings[39]. In 1958, Kupperman and colleagues conducted a prospective study, noting that androgens improved physical energy, libido and *joie de vivre*[40]. Further studies in the 1980s and 1990s have confirmed the findings of these early studies and provided information concerning hormonal effects on desire and arousal.

In 1985 Sherwin and co-workers published the results of a prospective study of surgically menopausal patients, showing that sexual drive correlated with testosterone levels, but frequency of sex activity or orgasm did not, suggesting that androgens primarily affect motivation[16]. Other studies gave further weight to the impact of testosterone on mood, well-being and sexual motivation in naturally and surgically menopausal women (Figures 3 and 4). Naturally menopausal women with mild-to-moderate vasomotor symptoms received esterified estrogens alone or with methyltestosterone over 12 weeks. The combined regimens, compared with other treatments, generally provided better relief of somatic symptoms. This study also noted that the lower-dose estrogen–androgen regimen (esterified estrogens 0.625 mg/day, plus methyltestosterone 1.25 mg/day) provided relief equal to that of the higher-dose regimen: esterified estrogens 1.25 mg/day plus methyltestosterone 2.5 mg/day. This finding further underscores the previously discussed importance of SHBG levels in determining the bioavailability of estrogen to target tissues. The addition of an androgenic component reduced SHBG levels, permitting a lower estrogen dose to be utilized with equal effectiveness[43].

Sarrel and co-workers in 1998 studied 20 naturally and surgically postmenopausal women who complained of decreased libido on traditional HRT. After a 2-month wash-out period, they were placed on either esterified estrogens or an esterified estrogen–methyltestosterone regimen. The combination group had a significant increase in sexual arousal and interest, as well as an increase in frequency of coitus[41] (see Figure 3).

More recently, Shifrin and colleagues reported on transdermal testosterone treatment in women with impaired sexual function after oophorectomy[17]. Seventy-five women, aged 31–56 years, received CEE (at least 0.625 mg/day) and, randomly, placebo or one of two dose levels of testosterone patches. Improvement in sexual function and psychological well-being was significantly demonstrated in the *older* women using the *higher*-dose patch. This interesting result in older versus younger patients may be a demonstration of the age differences in sexual problems; more physiological or anatomical and less psychological with increase in age.

Use of testosterone to treat sexual dysfunction

Most early papers demonstrating androgenic benefit utilized injections or pellets. Since that time, compounding pharmacists have formulated testosterone creams, gels and tablets that can be taken orally or used sublingually. However, their production is not uniform, they are not Food and Drug Administration (FDA) approved and academic studies of their efficacy are lacking. Many clinicians have tried creams used for vulvar dystrophies containing

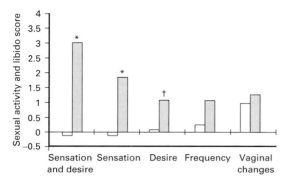

Figure 3 Estrogen–androgen therapy (shaded bars): improvement in sexual function over previous estrogen replacement therapy (white bars). $*p < 0.01$; $^{†}p \leq 0.05$. Adapted from reference 41

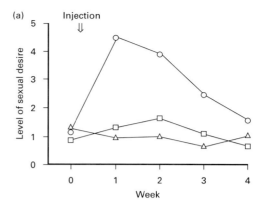

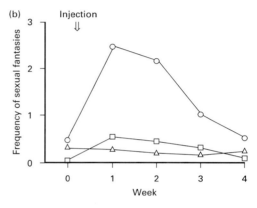

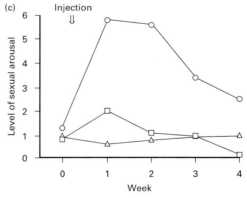

Figure 4 Mean level of sexual desire (a), frequency of sexual fantasies (b) and level of sexual arousal (c) following injection of an estrogen–androgen combination (circles), estrogen only (squares) or placebo (triangles). Adapted from reference 42

2% testosterone propionate. Others have tapered down the potency using micronized testosterone 0.5% up to 1% and rarely 2%. Creams were applied first on the inside of the forearms or thighs, while later paraclitoral use became common. Mixed results were commonplace, and the effect of rubbing the cream into the clitoris prior to intercourse, as some patients did, may have been nothing more than masturbatory pre-stimulation. Anecdotally, the creams seemed to work better paraclitorally in patients with sexual arousal disorder than in those with hypoactive sexual desire. Transdermal testosterone patches have been used in studies, but are not yet available. The only FDA-approved product in the USA is the combined esterified estrogen–methyltestosterone mentioned above, which is approved as an adjunct to estrogen replacement therapy for treatment of vasomotor symptoms as an alternative to increasing the estrogen dose. It is also used off-label to treat decline in sexual function or decreased capacity for arousal and orgasm[44]. Products formulated for use in men, such as the testosterone gel available in the USA, contain a much higher dosage than is suitable for women (Table 4).

Meanwhile, in Canada, Europe and Australia, more options have been available, including subcutaneous testosterone implants, intramuscular testosterone esters or nandrolone decanoate, and oral testosterone undecanoate. Some of these are either not available in the USA, or are carefully controlled, owing to their potential abuse by athletes.

Table 4 Androgen replacement therapy currently in use

	Dose range	Frequency	Route
Methyltestosterone* (in combination with esterified estrogens)	1.25–2.5 mg	daily	orally
Mixed testosterone esters	50–100 mg	4–6 weekly	intramuscularly
Testosterone implants	50 mg	3–6 monthly	subcutaneously
Transdermal testosterone patch[†]	150–300 µg	every 3.5 days	topically
Testosterone cream 1%[†]	5–10 mg	daily	topically
Testosterone undecanoate	40 mg	daily	orally
Nandrolone decanoate	50 mg	8–12 weekly	intramuscularly

*Currently available in the USA; [†]undergoing clinical trial

Studies on the use of DHEA, production of which is not regulated in the USA where, surprisingly, it is available over the counter, have shown an increase in sexual desire in androgen-deficient women. Improvement was demonstrated in energy level, well-being, sexual satisfaction and sexual function in pre- and postmenopausal women with low testosterone and DHEAS levels with adrenal insufficiency[45]. As there are no receptors for DHEA, these effects come from bioconversion to testosterone and/or estrogens[46].

Ongoing studies and clinical experience have shown that length of exposure is an important factor with respect to the successful use of androgens. While a small number of properly selected patients will respond in weeks, many will need to remain on the regimen for 3–4 months before any improvement in desire, libido, arousal, or orgasm may be noted.

Further effects of hormone replacement therapy

As mentioned above, oral estrogens in HRT as well as in OCs increase SHBG and can lead to decreased bioavailable estrogen and androgen, causing decreased libido, arousal, or orgasm[47]. It is for this reason that young women with premature ovarian failure might be best treated with an estrogen–androgen combination instead of OC therapy, to diminish the potential increase in SHBG. Other signs of increased SHBG include relapse of symptoms while still on HRT. Most

clinicians, when faced with a patient complaining of return of vasomotor symptoms, will increase the level of estrogen, which will allow only transient improvement, until SHBG levels rise further. Remember that the symptoms of too much estrogen can be the same as the symptoms of not enough estrogen, because of SHBG. A better choice would be to add an androgen or androgenic progestin, without changing the estrogen dosage, to decrease SHBG and increase levels of bioavailable testosterone and estrogen. A further option is to switch from oral to transdermal estrogen to decrease SHBG. When estrogen is given with a progestin, the effect on SHBG depends upon the type of progestin used. 19-Nortestosterone-derived progestins, such as norethindrone acetate, decrease SHBG levels, while derivatives of C-21 progesterone, such as MPA, do not significantly influence them[48].

Herbal therapies

The herbal or food additive market in the USA is a multibillion-dollar, totally unregulated industry. What is on the label is not necessarily in the jar, and what is in the jar is not necessarily on the label. Academic studies of efficacy are only beginning to appear in the literature. A smattering of papers have shown no statistical difference between St John's wort and placebo, ginseng and placebo, and dong quai and placebo. Some herbalists discount these studies because they explain that herbal therapy consists not of a single herb, but rather of a mixture of different herbs for each specific patient's problem; but patients purchase single herbal products over the counter, so the studies sample common practice. The good news is that academic programs around the USA have implemented alternative medicine sections or departments to learn about and evaluate the use of properly prepared herbal therapy, ultimately to incorporate this into Western medicine. Herbal products such as yohimbe and ginkgo biloba have been claimed to enhance desire, arousal and orgasm in both women and men. L-Arginine, an amino acid, has been touted as the natural Viagra®, due to its claimed ability to release nitric oxide, causing increased vasocongestion in the genitalia of both sexes[49]. Sex creams for paraclitoral use give a tingling clitoral sensation, mostly from the menthol in the cream, that is supposed to enhance orgasm. Oral breath mints can do the same. There is still much ground to cover on this issue.

Future therapies

There hardly exists a pharmaceutical company that does not have an androgen patch or gel in the 'pipeline' for women. Studies now in progress will give more conclusive results of the use of cream, sublingual and oral delivery systems.

Androgenic progestational agents, such as norethindrone acetate, a 19-nortestosterone derivative, have been used extensively in Europe in HRT regimens. Recently, their use has increased in the USA. The androgenic lineage of norethindrone acetate may demonstrate an effect on SHBG, desire and response to arousal similar to that seen with testosterone and methyltestosterone, although results of the few studies conducted to date have been inconclusive.

Tibolone, currently available in Europe and Australia, may gain FDA approval in the USA shortly. Taken orally, its metabolites have estrogenic, androgenic and progestational effects. The level of androgenic activity and its potential use for sexual dysfunction are under evaluation.

Sildenafil therapy in women is also undergoing evaluation. Preliminary findings demonstrate positive effects in appropriately selected women with normal testosterone levels. Improvements have been observed in the areas of sexual arousal and orgasm[50–52]. Studies are exploring both episodic as well as nightly use. Considering the common origin of female and male genitalia from the genital tubercle, it is anticipated that sildenafil will demonstrate benefit in some form or another in properly selected patients. Anecdotal reports of the use of crushed sildenafil in a cream base for paraclitoral use to increase clitoral vasocongestion have surfaced off-label as well.

Recently available in the USA, a clitoral suction device, modelled after a pump used before the advent of penile injections and sildenafil to produce and maintain erection in males, uses suction or negative pressure to increase vasocongestion and engorge the clitoris and paraclitoral tissues for enhanced arousal and orgasm[53].

Summary

The second modern sexual revolution has begun. The generation that brought free love to the college campuses in the 1960s and 1970s has reached chronological midlife and its members plan to continue their sexual ways. The problem is that their bodies do not function quite like they used to and they want answers and solutions. Sexual dysfunction can be understood only if sexual function is first clarified. Homologous structures retain homologous function, hence the broad similarities between the female and male physiology of sexual response. What drives sexuality, however, is quite different; intimacy, not orgasm, reigns in the female. Androgens are being intensively investigated for their place in the arena of sexuality as well as gaining importance peri- and postmenopausally, even though they begin to decline a decade earlier. 'Hormones, in their complex interplay, seem to control the intensity of libido and sexual behavior, rather than its direction, which is more dependent on motivational-affective and cognitive factors'[54]. Psychosocial and relationship issues influence sexual desire as much as, if not more than, physiology. Clinicians must avoid the 'easy-fix' pill trap and counsel or refer patients. True diagnostic guidelines are lacking, but much work is being carried out on this. Options for pharmacological therapy are expanding from hormones with varied delivery systems to vasoactive substances able to promote vasocongestion. Great progress has been made, but we have miles to go before we rest.

The best predictor of midlife sexuality is the state of the individual's earlier experience. With age, sexual interest persists, frequency of sexual activity diminishes and emphasis shifts from quantity to quality. Although sexual function may be compromised with age, gratification need not be sacrificed. The key question we need to ask our patients is, 'Are you or your partner troubled by this?'

References

1. Dennerstein L, Smith AM, Morse CA, Burger HG. Sexuality and the menopause. *J Psychosom Obstet Gynaecol* 1994;15:59–66
2. NFO Research, Inc. AARP/Modern Maturity Sexuality Study, 1999. Available at http://research.aarp.org/health/mmsexsurvey_1.html
3. Semmens JP, Wagner G. Estrogen deprivation and vaginal function in postmenopausal women. *J Am Med Assoc* 1982;248:445–8
4. Sarrel PM, Whitehead MI. Sex and menopause: defining the issues. *Maturitas* 1985;7:217–24
5. Marks LE. Sensory perception and ovarian secretions. In Naftolin F, DeCherney AH, Gutmann JN, Sarrel PM, eds. *Ovarian Secretions and Cardiovascular and Neurological Function*. New York: Raven Press, 1999:223–38
6. Berman JR, Berman LA, Werbin TJ, Flaherty EE, Leahy NM, Goldstein I. Clinical evaluation of female sexual function: effects of age and estrogen status on subjective and physiologic sexual responses. *Int J Impot Res* 1999;11(Suppl 1):S31–8
7. Shifren JL, Schiff I. The aging ovary. *J Womens Health Gend Based Med* 2000;9(Suppl 1):S3–7
8. Longcope C. The endocrinology of the menopause. In Lobo RA, ed. *Treatment of the Menopausal Woman: Basic and Clinical Aspects*. New York, NY: Raven, Ltd., 1994
9. Adashi EY. The climacteric ovary as a functional gonadotropin-driven androgen-producing gland. *Fertil Steril* 1994;62:20–7
10. Mushayandebvu T, Castracane VD, Gimpel T, Adel T, Santoro N. Evidence for diminished midcycle ovarian androgen production in older reproductive aged women. *Fertil Steril* 1996;65:721–3
11. Vermeulen A. The hormonal activity of the postmenopausal ovary. *J Clin Endocrinol Metab* 1976;42:247–53
12. Watts NB, Notelovitz M, Timmons MC, *et al.* Comparison of oral estrogens and estrogens plus androgen on bone mineral density, menopausal symptoms, and lipid–lipoprotein profiles in surgical menopause. *Obstet Gynecol* 1995;85:529–37
13. Davis SR, McCloud P, Strauss BJ, Burger H. Testosterone enhances estradiol's effects on postmenopausal bone density and sexuality. *Maturitas* 1995;21:227–36
14. Myers LS, Dixen J, Morrissette D, Carmichael M, Davidson JM. Effects of estrogen, androgen, and progestin on sexual psychophysiology and behavior in postmenopausal women. *J Clin Endocrinol Metab* 1990;70:1124–31
15. Greenblatt RB, Barfield WE, Garner JF, *et al.* Evaluation of an estrogen, androgen, and estrogen–androgen combination, and a placebo in the treatment of the menopause. *J Clin Endocrinol Metab* 1950;10:1547
16. Sherwin BB, Gelfand MM, Brender W. Androgen enhances sexual motivation in females; a prospective cross over study of sex steroid administration in the surgical menopause. *Psychosom Med* 1985;7:339–51
17. Shifrin JL, Braunstein GD, Simon JA, *et al.* Transdermal testosterone treatment in women with impaired sexual function after oopherectomy. *N Engl J Med* 2000;343:682–8
18. Davis SR. Androgen deficiency syndrome. *OBG Manage* 2000;May:4–6
19. Davis SR. Androgen treatment in women. *Med J Aust* 1999;170:545–9
20. Dunn JF, Nisula BC, Rodbard D. Transport of steroid hormones: binding of 21 endogenous steroids to both testosterone-binding globulin and corticosteroid-binding globulin in human plasma. *J Clin Endocrinol Metab* 1981;53:58–68

21. Stewart DE, Boydell K, Derzko C, Marshall V. Psychologic distress during the menopausal years in women attending a menopause clinic. *Int J Psychiatry Med* 1992;22:213–20

22. Leiblum J. *OBG Manage* 2000;May:10–13

23. Laumann EO, Paik A, Rosen RC. Sexual dysfunction in the United States: prevalence and predictors. *J Am Assoc* 1999;281:537–44

24. Masters WH, Johnson VE. *Human Sexual Repsonse*. Boston, MA: Little, Brown, 1966

25. Barash DP, Lipton JE. *The Myth of Monogamy*. New York: WH Freeman, 2001

26. Altman AM, Ashner L. *Making Love the Way We Used To...or Better; Secrets to Satisfying Midlife Sexuality*. Chicago: NTC/Contemporary Publishing, 2001

27. Kravitz HM, Haywood TW, Kelly J, Liles S, Cavanaugh JL Jr. Medroxyprogesterone and paraphiles: do testosterone levels matter? *Bull Am Acad Psychiatry Law* 1996;24:73–83

28. Weiner DN, Rosen RC. Medications and their impact. In Sipski ML, Alexander CJ, eds. *Sexual Function in People with Disability and Chronic Illness*. Gaithersberg, MD: Aspen Publishers, 1997:85–118

29. Hasson HM. Cervical removal at hysterectomy for benign disease: risks and benefits. *J Reprod Med* 1993;38:781–90

30. Rhodes JC, Kjerulff KH, Langenberg PW, Guzinski GM. Hysterectomy and sexual functioning. *J Am Med Assoc* 1999;282:1934–41

31. Basson R, Berman J, Burnett A, *et al*. Report of the International Consensus Development Conference on Female Sexual Dysfunction: definitions and classifications. *J Urol* 2000;163:888–93

32. Sarrel PM. Sexuality and menopause. *Obstet Gynecol*. 1990;75(Suppl 4):26S–30S; discussion 31S–35S

33. Chetkowski RJ, Meldrum DR, Steingold KA, *et al*. Biologic effects of transdermal estradiol. *N Engl J Med* 1986;314:1615–20

34. Sherwin BB. The impact of different doses of estrogen and progestin on mood and sexual behavior in postmenopausal women. *J Clin Endocrinol Metab* 1991;72:336–43

35. Fitzpatrick LA, Pace C, Wiita B. Comparison of regimens containing oral micronized progesterone or medroxyprogesterone acetate on quality of life in postmenopausal women: a cross-sectional survey. *J Womens Health Gend Based Med* 2000;9:381–7

36. Holst J, Backstrom T, Hammarback S, von Schoultz B. Progesterone addition during oestrogen replacement therapy – effects on vasomotor symptoms and mood. *Maturitas* 1989;11:13–20

37. Zhou J, Ng S, Adesanya-Tamuiga O, *et al*. Testosterone inhibits estrogen-induced mammary epithelial proliferation and suppresses estrogen receptor expression. *FASEB J* 2000;14:1725–30

38. Mor G, Eliza M, Song J, *et al*. 17α-Methyl testosterone is a competitive inhibitor of aromatase activity in Jar choriocarcinoma cells and macrophage-like THP-1 cells in culture. *J Steroid Biochem Molec Biol* 2001;79:239–46

39. Birnberg CH, Kurzrok R. Low-dosage androgen–estrogen therapy in the older age group. *J Am Geriatr Soc* 1955;3:656

40. Kupperman HS, Wetchler BB, Blatt MHG. Contemporary therapy of the menopausal syndrome. *J Am Med Assoc* 1959;171:1627

41. Sarrel P, Dobay B, Wiita B. Estrogen and estrogen–androgen replacement in postmenopausal women dissatisfied with estrogen-only therapy. Sexual behavior and neuroendocrine responses. *J Reprod Med* 1998;43:847–56

42. Sherwin BB, Gelfand MM. The role of androgen in the maintenance of sexual functioning in oophorectomized women. *Psychosom Med* 1987;49:397–409

43. Simon J, Klaiber E, Wiita B, Bowen A, Yang HM. Differential effects of estrogen–androgen and estrogen-only therapy on vasomotor symptoms, gonadotropin secretion, and endogenous androgen bioavailability in postmenopausal women. *Menopause* 1999;6:138–46

44. Davis SR. The clinical use of androgens in female sexual disorders. *J Sex Marital Ther* 1998;24:153–63

45. Guay AT. Advances in the management of androgen deficiency in women. *Med Asp Hum Sex* 2001;1:32–8

46. Arlt W, Callies F, Allolio B. DHEA replacement in women with adrenal insufficiency – pharmacokinetics, bioconversion and clinical effects on well-being, sexuality and cognition. *Endocr Res* 2000;26:505–11

47. Mathur RS, Landgrebe SC, Moody LO, Semmens JP, Williamson HO. The effect of estrogen treatment on plasma concentrations of steroid hormones, gonadotropins, prolactin and sex hormone-binding globulin in post-menopausal women. *Maturitas* 1985;7:129–33

48. Stomati M, Hartmann B, Spinetti A, *et al*. Effects of hormonal replacement therapy on plasma sex hormone-binding globulin, androgen and insulin-like growth factor-1 levels in postmenopausal women. *J Endocrinol Invest* 1996;19:535–41

49. Chen J, Wollman Y, Chernichovsky T, Iaina A, Sofer M, Matzkin H. Effect of oral administration of high-dose nitric oxide donor

L-arginine in men with organic erectile dysfunction: results of a double-blind, randomized, placebo-controlled study. *BJU Int* 1999; 83:269–73

50. Agnello C. Premenopausal women affected by sexual arousal disorder treated with sildenafil: a double-blind, cross-over, placebo-controlled study. *Br J Obstet Gynaecol* 2001;108:623–8

51. Salerian AJ, Deibler WE, Vittone BJ, *et al*. Sildenafil for psychotropic-induced sexual dysfunction in 31 women and 61 men. *J Sex Marital Ther* 2000;26:133–40

52. Kaplan SA, Reis RB, Kohn IJ, *et al*. Safety and efficacy of sildenafil in postmenopausal women with sexual dysfunction. *Urology* 1999; 53:481–6

53. Wilson SK, Delk JR 2nd, Billups KL. Treating symptoms of female sexual arousal disorder with the Eros-Clitoral Therapy Device. *J Gend Specif Med* 2001;4:54–8

54. Graziottin A. Loss of libido in the postmenopause. *Menopausal Med* 2000;8:9–12

Symptoms of the perimenopause

7

L. Dennerstein and J. Guthrie

Introduction

Studies of middle-aged women suggest that they are highly symptomatic[1,2] and therefore likely to present to primary care services. The midlife years of 45–55 coincide with those of the menopausal transition. Important clinical questions to determine are which symptoms are the most prevalent in midlife, which symptoms relate to the hormonal changes underlying the menopause and which symptoms reflect aging. The role of psychosocial and lifestyle factors in determining women's experience of symptoms is also of interest to clinicians.

Measuring symptoms

Conflicting findings as to the etiology of symptoms in midlife reflect some of the methodological difficulties inherent in menopause research as well as specific issues pertaining to the measurement of symptoms. There are inter- and intracultural differences in symptom reporting. Kaufert and Syrotuik[3] described how stereotypes held by differing social and cultural groups act as a framework within which an individual can select, organize and label experience. Potential biases that can occur during the ascertainment of symptom data include both interviewer bias in the phrasing of questions and specification bias if the variable under study is not well specified to the full understanding of the subject. The length of the recall period can lead to further inaccuracy of data and this has varied widely in the published literature. Another source of error in analyzing observational study data on the determinants of symptom experiences is that of confounding, which necessitates the use of multivariate analytic methods to control for the influence of the various factors that can affect an outcome.

A major issue is that of the symptom measure utilized, and its validity and reliability for the cultural group studied. The standard method used for collecting information on the prevalence and severity of symptoms has been a checklist of symptoms, but the checklist in itself introduces a number of biases including the problem of elicitation. For example, Wright[4], interviewing women of the Navajo tribe, found that virtually all respondents reported no bodily changes since the menopause in relation to open-ended questions, but most responded positively to symptoms in the checklist. Holte[5] noted that the sounder the methodology, the lower the prevalence of symptoms. The Melbourne Women's Midlife Health Project found that moving the position of a symptom in a symptom checklist significantly affected its reported prevalence[6]. When frequency and bothersomeness of a complaint are included, the reporting rate goes down further[5]. For example, irritability was reported by 57% of premenopausal women as being present occasionally but only 10% of the same women reported that it was there frequently. The presence of symptoms 'occasionally' does not indicate their impact on the woman and may not be clinically relevant or indicative of treatment needs. Porter and co-workers[7] assessed the impact and prevalence of symptoms in a Scottish postal survey of 6096 women aged 45–54 years. Fifty-seven per cent of the cohort had experienced a hot flash but only 22% said that it had been a problem. Similar disparity existed for night sweats (55% and 24%) and dry vagina (34% and 14%). Only 4% had experienced none of the symptoms.

The most frequently used checklist has been based on a numerical summation of 11 menopausal complaints, the Kupperman Menopausal Index[8], derived from clinical experience in New York in the 1950s. The index was a combination of self-report and physician ratings. The index included 11 symptoms rated on a four-point scale: vasomotor, paresthesia, insomnia, nervousness, melancholia, vertigo, weakness (fatigue), arthralgia and myalgia, headaches, palpitations and formication. In a critical review, Alder[9] noted that terms were ill-defined, categories included overlapping scores and scores were summed without being based on independent factors. Symptoms seemed to be arbitrarily selected – omitted were measures of vaginal dryness, dyspareunia and breast tenderness. Kupperman and co-workers[8] and, the following year, Blatt and Wiesbader[10] described a modification that allowed for some symptoms to be weighted more than others. Weighting was used without statistical justification. Later investigators, such as Neugarten and Kraines[11], extended the list to 28 symptoms but found that only nine of these distinguished menopausal women from those at other developmental phases. These authors, and many since, arbitrarily categorized groups of symptoms. Greene[12] was the first to use factor analysis as the basis for categorizing symptoms into three factors, which he termed vasomotor, somatic and psychological. However, Greene's study contained a number of flaws. Although his 30-symptom list was constructed from the scale of Neugarten and Kraines[11] he failed to include breast pain, somewhat curiously, as Neugarten and Kraines had found this symptom to be associated with menopausal women. Furthermore, he did not include symptoms of vaginal atrophy. Nor were these symptoms included in a later amended 20-item list[13].

Whether psychological complaints vary with the menopausal transition has been a key question, yet the capacity of most symptom checklists adequately to measure psychological morbidity is unknown[3]. In a Manitoba study[3], symptoms measuring psychological morbidity had to conform to scales used by psychological epidemiologists, and concurrent validity was sought. The symptom checklist was not restricted to items with an association with the menopause but was embedded in an 18-item general symptom list adapted from one used in a community health survey. The 11 symptoms forming the menopausal index were derived from the International Health Foundation studies (hot flash, night sweats, dizziness, rapid heart beat, 'pins and needles' in hands and feet, tiredness, irritability, headaches, depression, nervous tension and insomnia). Interestingly, the list did not include vaginal atrophy symptoms, yet the International Health Foundation list was chosen as a 'succinct summary of the core symptoms as described in the clinical literature'. Subsequent analysis found four factors. Hot flashes and night sweats were grouped together as a separate factor and five symptoms were loaded on to a psychological factor. These were five of the six factors in the International Health Foundation arbitrary classification of 'symptoms of the nervous system'. A strong association was found between the five psychological symptoms and the two standardized measures of psychological morbidity used for concurrent validity.

Greene[13] compared the findings of seven-factor analytic studies. Despite different methodologies and sampling he found that vasomotor symptoms (hot flashes, night sweats) always formed a separate cluster, totally independent of other symptoms. There was also agreement that a number of symptoms cluster together to form a general somatic or perhaps psychosomatic factor: pressure or tightness in the head or body, muscle and joint pains, numb/tingling feelings, headaches, feeling dizzy or faint, breathing difficulties, and loss of feeling in hands or feet. A further group of symptoms clustered together to form a psychological factor, which in some studies can be subdivided into anxiety and depression.

The Melbourne Women's Midlife Health Project

The Melbourne Women's Midlife Health Project (MWMHP) has used a number of strategies to overcome these problems in study design. These include a strictly random, community-based sample of 2001 Australian-born women, residing in Melbourne, aged between 45 and 55 years (71% response rate)[2]. The women were identified for the baseline study from the general population using random telephone digital dialling; describing the study as a general health survey, so that bias caused by stereotypic response to menopause was lessened; collecting information on bothersome symptoms experienced in the past 2 weeks so that the problem of recall bias was minimized; utilizing a baseline age range that encompassed the menopausal transition, i.e. 45–55 years; longer follow-up (currently 9 years from baseline); and prospective collection of data on health outcomes, menstrual status and any hormone usage, so that phase of the natural menopausal transition can be adequately determined. Questionnaires carefully constructed by Kaufert and McKinlay and colleagues and used in cross-sectional and longitudinal studies in North America[3,14] were used to measure symptoms and other variables. We previously reported cross-sectional analysis of baseline interview data including factor analysis of the symptom checklist[2]. Hormone levels were not assessed at baseline but were introduced into the longitudinal study, which involved annual interviews and collection of blood for hormone estimation[6].

Prevalence of symptoms in middle-aged women

The symptoms reported by middle-aged women in the MWMHP baseline cohort of 2001 women are shown in Table 1. The most frequently reported symptom was that of aches/stiff joints (reported by 52% of the cohort), whilst hot flashes were eighth on the list (29% of cohort). Table 1 reports the percentage of women reporting each symptom as bothersome in the prior 2 weeks.

Table 1 Percentage of women ($n = 2001$) who were bothered by symptoms in the previous 2 weeks

Symptom	Percentage
Aches or stiff joints	51.5
Lack of energy	43.2
Nervous tension	41.8
Backaches	40.0
Trouble sleeping	37.9
Headaches	35.0
Feeling sad or downhearted	31.0
Hot flashes	29.0
Difficulty in concentrating	25.0
Tingling/pins and needles in hands and feet	21.7
Swelling of parts of the body	20.1
Shortness of breath	16.9
Sore throat	15.4
Problems with control of urine	15.2
Diarrhea or constipation	12.7
Upset stomach	12.2
Rapid heart beat	11.7
Persistent cough	9.5
Dizzy spells	9.3
Cold sweats	8.2
Loss of appetite	5.4
Bladder infection problems	2.3

Symptom change, gender and age

One method of determining whether symptoms are related to the menopause or to aging is to compare prevalence results for men and women. Two studies have compared symptom checklist results for men and women of different age groups using lists from general practices. Results were presented by age groups rather than by menopausal status. Bungay and associates[15], in a UK postal survey, found that four different patterns occurred by age and sex. Peaks of prevalence of flashing and sweating were closely associated with the mean age of the menopause. Less impressive peaks of minor mental symptoms were associated with an age just preceding the mean age of menopause. Complaints about aching breasts, irritability and low backache diminished after menopause. Male and female curves were parallel for: loss of appetite, crawling or tingling sensations on the skin, headaches, difficulty with intercourse, indigestion, constipation, diarrhea, shortness of breath, coldness of hands and feet, dryness of skin, dryness of hair, aching muscles, aching joints, feelings of panic, feelings of depression and stinging on passing water.

A Dutch national study[16] of the symptoms in the Kupperman index of men and women aged over 25 years reported female/male ratios for each symptom. Only transpiration (excessive sweating) showed a significant increase at age 45–54 compared with younger age groups and then remained raised. No other symptom showed a significant increase in the age group of 45–54 including the GHQ score of mental health.

Symptom change and the menopause

There is consensus about the marked temporal relationship of vasomotor symptoms to the menopause[17]. These begin to increase in the perimenopause, reaching a peak within 1–2 years of the final menstrual period (FMP)[18] and remain elevated for up to 10 years[19–21]. McKinlay and colleagues[22], in a follow-up study over 4 years of 1178 premenopausal women, found increasing hot flashes (10% in early premenopause, 30% in early perimenopause, increasing to 50% of women 1 year prior to the FMP – coinciding with late perimenopause), with reports of hot flashes starting to decline significantly 2 years after the FMP, and reaching 20% of women 4 years after the FMP. Thus, hot flashes are not the most frequent symptoms reported, nor are they pathognomonic of the menopause, being reported by younger menstruating women. A number of studies have shown an association between hot flashes and night sweats[23], and some show an association between these vasomotor symptoms and insomnia[24].

Women who had an artificially induced menopause were more likely still to be flashing than were naturally menopausal women and to report more symptoms[24]. Only a few studies included dryness of the vagina. Oldenhave and Jaszmann[21] reported that dry vagina increased in the peri- to postmenopause with a slight decrease > 10 years

postmenopause which may be explained by lack of a partner. This complaint is related to hot flash reporting. There was less consistency regarding other symptoms. A number of cross-sectional studies, including the two Ede studies[19,21], reported a small but transient increase in non-vasomotor symptoms in the perimenopause. It is not clear whether any increase in such symptoms is due to distress caused by vasomotor symptoms. A number of other studies, including recent longitudinal studies using validated mood scales, have not found an association between mood and menopausal status.

The MWMHP analyzed data from those women who were premenopausal at baseline and, by the end of the seventh year of follow-up, reported three or more months of amenorrhea. Each woman contributed 7 years of data, or, if she experienced a surgical menopause (through hysterectomy, bilateral oophorectomy, endometrial or iatrogenic ablation) or took hormone therapy during the study, only those observations taken prior to this medical intervention were analyzed.

Using results obtained from the longitudinal phase of the MWMHP, we report the proportion of women experiencing a particular symptom as bothersome in the previous 2 weeks for each category of menopausal status (Table 2). Note that the number of women available for analysis decreased in the peri- and postmenopausal groups, owing to the increasing numbers of women taking up hormone replacement therapy (HRT) as the study progressed, as well as other reasons for exclusion.

Means of symptom severity scores were then calculated (μ_1) for each woman in the pre- and early perimenopausal years and these were compared (using paired t tests) with mean symptom severity scores (μ_2) for the late peri- and postmenopausal years. Menopausal categories were grouped in this way, as previous analyses had identified the 'late perimenopause' as the phase of maximum change in levels of follicle stimulating hormone (FSH) and estradiol[25], and the phase that best discriminated the dataset of health

Table 2 Percentage of the sample reporting a symptom in the past 2 weeks by menopausal category. From reference 6, with permission

| Symptom | Premenopausal (n = 172) | Early perimenopausal (n = 148) | Late perimenopausal (n = 106) | Postmenopausal | | |
				1 year (n = 72)	2 years (n = 54)	3 years (n = 31)
Dizzy spells	11.6	13.5	11.3	13.9	13.0	25.8
Lack of energy*	42.4	43.2	42.5	37.5	42.6	41.9
Diarrhea/constipation	11.6	17.6	16.0	19.4	7.4	19.4
Persistent cough	7.6	12.2	15.1	13.9	7.4	3.2
Feeling sad/downhearted	25.6	26.4	37.7	27.8	31.5	25.8
Backaches	30.2	33.8	34.0	34.7	37.0	38.7
Upset stomach	12.2	14.2	9.4	12.5	13.0	22.6
Headaches/migraines	38.4	37.2	35.8	36.1	31.5	41.9
Cold sweats	1.7	5.4	7.5	2.8	1.9	6.5
Aches or stiff joints	41.3	47.3	52.8	52.8	57.4	45.2
Shortness of breath at rest	5.9	2.2	5.2	5.6	3.7	0
Tingling in hands/feet	17.4	23.6	19.8	19.4	24.1	29.0
Sore throat	13.4	16.2	15.1	9.7	9.3	12.9
Trouble sleeping	30.8	31.8	37.7	37.5	42.6	45.2
Chest pain on exertion	1.5	2.2	0	2.8	0	3.2
Loss of appetite	2.9	6.1	4.7	2.8	1.9	6.5
Swelling in parts of the body	18.0	27.0	18.9	13.9	18.5	19.4
Difficulty in concentrating	20.9	20.9	18.9	27.8	20.4	25.8
Shortness of breath on exertion	22.1	18.3	19.8	12.5	27.8	16.1
Nervous tension	32.6	29.7	39.6	30.6	31.5	25.8
Problems with urine control	17.4	12.2	14.2	13.9	25.9	16.1
Bladder infection problems	1.2	1.4	0.9	2.8	1.9	3.2
Discomfort on passing urine	1.9	0.7	1.9	2.8	0	3.2
Rapid heart beat	8.7	9.5	13.2	11.1	5.6	9.7
Hot flashes	9.9	14.9	41.5	41.7	40.7	51.6
Night sweats	10.3	13.5	30.2	34.7	24.1	41.9
Dry vagina	2.9	4.3	20.8	25.0	31.5	47.4
Troublesome vaginal discharge	3.7	2.7	2.8	2.8	1.9	0
Dry eyes	3.0	14.3	12.8	18.8	20.4	25.8
Dry nose or mouth	12.1	7.1	14.0	17.4	9.3	16.1
Weight gain or loss (> 3 kg)	0.9	1.4	0.9	2.8	0	3.2
Skin irritation (crawling/dryness)	10.3	19.6	21.7	11.1	14.8	12.9
Breast soreness/tenderness	33.0	33.9	12.8	7.2	3.7	6.5

*Lack of energy may give unreliable results – change in sequence order from the 5th year of follow-up

outcomes. Geometric mean hormone levels of estradiol and FSH by menopausal phase for the present sample are shown in Figure 1.

For those symptoms that showed significant change in the above analysis, further analysis was carried out in order to differentiate age effects from those due to change in menopausal status. Sample proportions (reported with 95% confidence intervals (CI)) were compared across the following

menopausal categories: premenopause (the year prior to the first report of change in menstrual frequency), early perimenopause (the first reported year of change in menstrual frequency), late perimenopause (the first reported year of amenorrhea (3–11 months)), and postmenopause (+1, +2 and +3) years after the FMP.

Figure 2 summarizes the results when mean severity scores within individuals for each

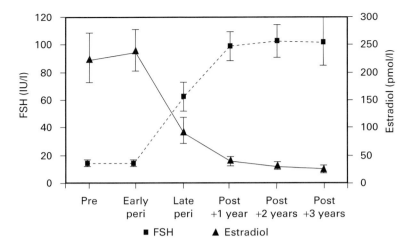

Figure 1 Geometric means (± 95% confidence intervals) of hormone levels by menopausal status ($n = 172$). FSH, follicle stimulating hormone. From reference 6, with permission

symptom before late perimenopause were compared with mean severity scores obtained from late perimenopause and thereafter. Symptoms are listed in increasing order of change, where 0 indicates no change. Significant differences were found where the 95% CI did not cross the 0 line. It can be seen that severity scores for breast soreness were significantly reduced in the late perimenopause and postmenopause compared with breast soreness scores obtained in the premenopause and early perimenopause. Symptom severity of insomnia, dry vagina, night sweats and hot flashes were all significantly increased in the late perimenopause and postmenopause. No other symptom showed any significant change with menopausal status.

In order to differentiate the effect of aging from that of menopause, sample proportions (± 95% confidence intervals CI) were compared across the six categories for menopausal status. The following symptoms were found to increase significantly between the early and the late perimenopause: hot flashes (+27%), night sweats (+17%) and dry vagina (+17%), while breast soreness/tenderness decreased significantly (–21%). The increase in insomnia at the late perimenopause (+6%) was not significant. Insomnia thus seems to be related more to aging than to menopausal status.

Risk factors for developing menopausal symptoms

Cross-sectional studies have explored the association between symptom experience and a large range of other factors. In keeping with other studies from Australia, North America, Scandinavia and Europe, our baseline Melbourne study found lower symptom experience in the midlife years to be associated with increasing years of education, better self-rated health, the use of fewer non-prescription medications, absence of chronic conditions, a low level of interpersonal stress, absence of premenstrual complaints, absence of current smoking, exercise at least once per week and positive attitudes to aging and to menopause[2]. Vasomotor symptoms have been found to be associated with decreasing estradiol[26,27], increasing FSH[26] and decreasing exercise levels[2,28,29]. More detailed studies of exercise have not found beneficial effects on troubling symptoms[30].

Longitudinal population-based studies are best able to establish the likely relationship between experience of symptoms and psychosocial and lifestyle factors. The Massachusetts Women's Health Study found that prior physical and psychological symptoms explained physical symptoms, while psychological

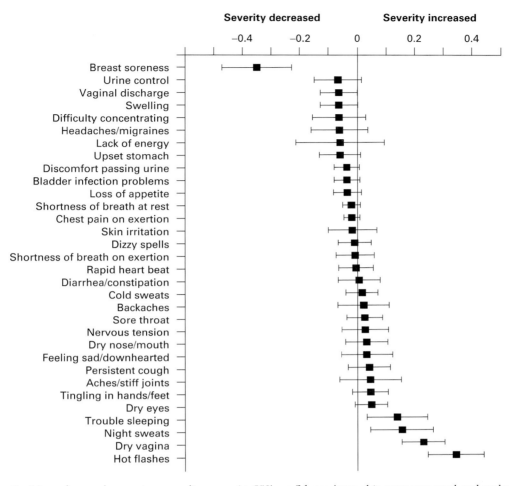

Figure 2   Mean changes in symptom severity scores (± 95% confidence intervals): premenopausal and early perimenopausal scores compared with late perimenopausal and postmenopausal scores. From reference 6, with permission

symptoms were explained by low education and perceived health[14]. A further analysis of the 454 women from this sample who were premenopausal at baseline and postmenopausal by the sixth follow-up found that variables related to a greater frequency of vasomotor reporting included a longer perimenopause, more symptoms reported prior to menopause, lower education and more negative attitudes to menopause prior to menopause[31]. Symptom bothersomeness was related to a greater frequency of vasomotor symptom reporting, smoking and being divorced. Variables that predicted

consultations were greater frequency and bothersomeness of symptoms, higher education and greater health-care utilization[31]. Women with negative attitudes to menopause were more likely subsequently to experience bothersome symptoms[32].

A British study[33] found that women who had experienced an early natural menopause had a strongly raised risk of vasomotor symptoms (hot flashes or night sweats), sexual difficulties (vaginal dryness or difficulties with intercourse) and trouble sleeping. However, there was little or no excess risk of other somatic or psychological symptoms. In contrast, all types of symptoms were more common among women who had a hysterectomy or were users of HRT. Using prospective data collected when the women were 36, symptom reporting was predicted by low education, stressful lives, or a previous history of poor physical and psychological health. Adjustment for these factors in a logistic regression model did not affect the relations between symptoms and current menopausal status. For vasomotor symptoms, postmenopausal women had an adjusted odds ratio of 4.7 (95% CI 2.6–8.5) and perimenopausal women had an adjusted odds ratio of 2.6 (95% CI 1.9–3.5) compared with premenopausal women. Corresponding adjusted odds ratios for sexual difficulties were 3.9 (95% CI 2.1–7.1) and 2.2 (95% CI 1.4–3.2), and for insomnia were 3.4 (95% CI 1.9–6.2) and 1.5 (95% CI 1.1–2.0).

A postal survey of men and women aged between 49 and 55 years, registered with a London general practice[34], found no gender differences in reporting of self-rated health, life satisfaction and health-related quality of life, although women reported more physical problems. Menopausal status was not significantly related to life satisfaction or to health-related quality of life. Significant predictors of health-related quality of life were serious illness, and employment and marital status. Sample size was relatively small in this study (189), response rate was only 47% and the age range may have meant that most women were already in the menopausal transition.

Using structural modelling of data from the first 6 years of follow-up of the MWMHP, the presence of bothersome symptoms was found to affect well-being adversely[35]. Repeated measure multivariate analysis of covariance also found that bothersome symptoms adversely impacted on negative mood[35].

Predictors of menopausal symptoms

The MWMHP used logistic regression to compare women who developed the symptom in the late perimenopause with those women who did not. Hot flashes were predicted by a history of premenstrual complaints ($p < 0.05$), increased levels of lifetime smoking ($p < 0.05$) and increased levels of FSH ($p < 0.01$). The only variable predicting night sweats in the late perimenopause was log(estradiol) ($p < 0.05$). A decrease (or large decline) in estradiol levels was associated with an increase in the reporting of night sweats. The only variable to be retained in the model predicting dry vagina in the late perimenopause was level of education. More than 12 years of education was associated with decreased reporting of dry vagina.

Three variables were retained in the multivariate model predicting insomnia in the late perimenopause. Decreased well-being ($p < 0.01$), agreement with the belief that 'women with many interests in their lives hardly notice menopause' ($p < 0.05$) and the presence of hot flashes ($p < 0.01$) were associated with increased reporting of insomnia.

Implications for clinicians

By midlife the majority of women report bothersome symptoms when questioned, yet only a few of these relate to the hormonal changes of the menopausal transition. These are the vasomotor symptoms of hot flashes and night sweats, the atrophic symptoms of dryness in the vagina and associated dyspareunia, insomnia (as sleep is affected by vasomotor symptoms as well as aging and mood) and breast tenderness, which declines significantly as women reach the later phases of the menopausal transition. A reduction in breast tenderness associated with several missed or skipped menses and increased vasomotor symptoms and FSH may indicate to the clinician that the woman is in the late menopausal transition and her final menses will probably occur within the next year. Vasomotor and atrophic symptoms are responsive to HRT, which could also be expected to improve insomnia related to night-time occurrence of vasomotor symptoms. Healthy lifestyles, increased knowledge and positive attitudes to menopause and to aging will help prevent exacerbation of endocrine-related symptoms by psychosocial factors.

References

1. Avis NE, Kaufert PA, Lock M, McKinlay SM, Vass K. The evolution of menopausal symptoms. *Baillière's Clin Endocrinol Metab* 1993; 7:17–32

2. Dennerstein L, Smith AMA, Morse CA, *et al.* Menopausal symptomatology in Australian women. *Med J Aust* 1993;159:232–6

3. Kaufert P, Syrotuik J. Symptom reporting at the menopause. *Soc Sci Med [E]* 1981;15:173–84

4. Wright A. On the calculation of climacteric symptoms. *Maturitas* 1981;3:55–63

5. Holte A. Prevalence of climacteric complaints in a representative sample of middle-aged women in Oslo, Norway. *J Psychosom Obstet Gynaecol* 1991;12:303–17

6. Dennerstein L, Dudley E, Hopper J, Guthrie JR, Burger H. A prospective population-based study of menopausal symptoms. *Obstet Gynecol* 2000;96:351–8

7. Porter M, Penney G, Russell D, Russell E, Templeton A. A population-based survey of women's experience of the menopause. *Br J Obstet Gynaecol* 1996;103:1025–8

8. Kupperman H, Blatt M, Wiesbader H, Togashi S. Use of the amenorrhoea and menopausal index in the clinical evaluation of estrogenic compounds. *Fed Proc* 1952;11:365

9. Alder E. The Blatt–Kupperman menopausal index; a critique. *Maturitas* 1998;29:19–24

10. Blatt M, Wiesbader H, Kuppermann HS. Vitamin E and climacteric syndrome. *Arch Intern Med* 1953;91:792–9

11. Neugarten B, Kraines RJ. Menopausal symptoms in women of various ages. *Psychosom Med* 1965;27:266–73

12. Greene J. A factor analytic study of climacteric symptoms. *J Psychosom Res* 1976;20:425–30

13. Greene J. Constructing a standard climacteric scale. *Maturitas* 1998;29:25–31

14. McKinlay J, McKinlay S, Brambilla D. The relative contributions of endocrine changes and social circumstances to depression in mid-aged women. *J Health Soc Behav* 1987;28:345–63

15. Bungay G, Vessey M, McPherson C, *et al.* Study of symptoms in middle life with special reference to the menopause. *Br Med J* 1980;281: 181–3

16. Van Hall E, Verdel M, van der Velden J. 'Perimenopausal' complaints in women and men: a comparative study. *J Women's Health* 1994;3:45–9

17. Greene J. The cross-sectional legacy: an introduction to longitudinal studies of the climacteric. *Maturitas* 1992;14:95–101

18. Holte A. Prevalence of climacteric complaints in a representative sample of middle-aged women in Oslo, Norway. *J Psychosom Obstet Gynaecol* 1991;12:303–17

19. Jaszmann L, van Lith N, Zaat J. The perimenopausal symptoms: the statistical analysis of a survey. Part A. *Med Gynecol Sociol* 1969;4: 268–77

20. Ballinger C. Psychiatric morbidity and the menopause; screening of general population sample. *Br Med J* 1975;3:344–6

21. Oldenhave A, Jaszmann L. The climacteric: absence or presence of hot flushes and their relation to other complaints. In Schonbaum E, ed. *The Climacteric Hot Flush. Progress in Basic Clinical Pharmacology*. Basel: Karger, 1991;6:6–39

22. McKinlay S, Brambilla D, Posner J. The normal menopause transition. *Maturitas* 1992;14: 103–15

23. McKinlay S, Jeffereys M. The menopausal syndrome. *Br J Prev Soc Med* 1974;28:108–15

24. Thompson B, Hart S, Durno D. Menopausal age and symptomatology in a general practice. *J Biosoc Sci* 1973;5:71–82

25. Burger HG, Dudley E, Groome N, *et al.* Prospectively measured levels of serum FSH, estradiol and the dimeric inhibins during the menopausal transition in a population-based cohort of women. *J Clin Endocrinol Metab* 1999;84:4025–30

26. Guthrie JR, Dennerstein L, Hopper JL, Burger HG. Hot flushes, menstrual status, and hormone levels in a population-based sample of midlife women. *Obstet Gynecol* 1996;88:437–42

27. Wilbur J, Miller A, Montgomery A, Chandler P. Sociodemographic characteristics, biological factors, and symptom reporting in midlife women. *Menopause* 1998;5:43–51

28. Ivarsson T, Spetz A, Hammar M. Physical exercise and vasomotor symptoms in postmenopausal women. *Maturitas* 1998;29:139–46

29. Collins A. Experience of symptoms during transition to menopause: a population-based longitudinal study. In *Proceedings of the 7th International Congress on the Menopause*, Stockholm. Carnforth, UK: Parthenon Publishing, 1993

30. Guthrie J, Smith A, Dennerstein L, Morse C. Physical activity and the menopause experience: a cross-sectional study. *Maturitas* 1995;20:71–80

31. Avis N, Crawford S, McKinlay S. Psychosocial, behavioral, and health factors related to menopause symptomatology. *Womens Health* 1997;3:103–20

32. Avis N, McKinlay S. A longitudinal analysis of women's attitudes toward the menopause: results from the Massachusetts Women's Health Study. *Maturitas* 1991;13:65–79

33. Kuh D, Wadsworth M, Hardy R. Women's health in midlife: the influence of the menopause, social factors and health in earlier life. *Br J Obstet Gynaecol* 1997;104:923–33

34. O'Dea I, Hunter M, Anjos S. Life satisfaction and health-related quality of life (SF-36) of middle aged men and women. *Climacteric* 1999;2:131–40

35. Dennerstein L, Lehert P, Burger H, Dudley E. Mood and the menopausal transition. *J Nerv Ment Disord* 1999;187:685–91

Bleeding patterns in perimenopausal women

8

S. R. Goldstein

Abnormal uterine bleeding, commonly encountered in gynecological practice, accounts for 20% of office visits[1] and almost 25% of gynecological operations[2]. The patient who presents with perimenopausal bleeding presents two distinct but important challenges for the clinician. The first is the exclusion of cancer or hyperplasia; the second is the annoyance as well as fear that the bleeding engenders.

Risks of cancer

The perimenopause is a relatively newly classified clinical entity, although women have endured its physiological challenges since antiquity. It is defined by The World Health Organization[3] as beginning 2–8 years preceding menopause and lasting up to 12 months after the final menses. The incidence of endometrial carcinoma increases with age. The rate of endometrial carcinoma in women aged 30–39 is 2.3/100 000; in women aged 35–39, it increases to 6.1/100 000; and in women aged 40–49 it is 36.2/100 000[4]. Recommendations from The American College of Obstetricians and Gynecologists are that, based on age alone, endometrial assessment to exclude cancer is indicated in any woman older than 35 who is suspected of having anovulatory uterine bleeding[5]. One study[6] of 433 women between 39 and menopause with any break in menstrual cyclicity revealed no carcinoma and an incidence of hyperplasia of 2.5% (11/433). Of these, five were in globally thickened endometria and six were contained within polyps.

Abnormal uterine bleeding can have a variety of menstrual patterns which by clinical experience have yielded empiric definitions. These include:

(1) Intermenstrual bleeding – bleeding between menstrual cycles;

(2) Metrorrhagia – irregular bleeding;

(3) Menorrhagia – excessive bleeding at regular intervals;

(4) Polymenorrhea – menstrual cycle interval less than 21 days;

(5) Oligomenorrhea – menstrual cycle interval longer than 37 days.

Often any abnormality of menstrual flow is assigned the term 'menometrorrhagia', so that it loses its meaning as an important historical clue to the etiology (Table 1). Ovulatory cycles are most likely to be regular in nature, although their variability is most commonly due to variations in the proliferative (follicular) phase. Metrorrhagia or intermenstrual bleeding is likely to represent dysfunctional anovulatory bleeding, although non-uterine causes (cervical or vaginal, inflammatory or neoplastic) must be excluded. Clearly, an antecedent pregnancy event must always be ruled out as well. Leiomyomata are quite common, especially in midlife women. The exact mechanism by which a leiomyoma results in abnormal uterine bleeding is not entirely clear, but certainly, those of the submucous variety are most frequently responsible. In addition, as uterine cavity size grows,

Table 1 Findings in perimenopausal patients with abnormal uterine bleeding

Reference	Normal cavity	Myoma	Polyps	Hyperplasia	Cancer	Other*
Indman ($n = 234$)[34]	41% ($n = 97$)	32% ($n = 75$)	20% ($n = 47$)	2% ($n = 5$)	1% ($n = 2$)	4% ($n = 8$)
Towbin *et al.* ($n = 149$)[35]	24% ($n = 35$)	33% ($n = 49$)	22% ($n = 33$)	4% ($n = 6$)	0% ($n = 0$)	17% ($n = 26$)
Goldstein *et al.* ($n = 433$)[6]	79% ($n = 341$)	5% ($n = 22$)[†]	13% ($n = 58$)	3% ($n = 11$)	0% ($n = 0$)	0% ($n = 0$)

*Includes polyp and myoma, 'adenomyosis'; [†]submucous myoma, although 34% had sonographic evidence of any leiomyomata

with some, but not all enlarging fibroids, the concurrent menorrhagia may simply be the result of an increase in the surface area of the endometrium. The same is true of the increasing uterine size seen with increasing parity.

Physiological changes of the perimenopause

The first clinically evident sign of perimenopause is a break in cyclicity in women with a previously regular menstrual cycle pattern. However, for many women, menstrual cycle patterns vary greatly[7]. Intermenstrual intervals often shorten, on the one hand, but may become markedly irregular as well[8]. This may result in long cycles being interspersed with very short ones[9]. For many women the cycle may shorten by 3–7 days as the result of a shortened follicular phase, i.e. ovulation taking place prior to day 14[10]. Some women will have irregular spotting while others will skip several cycles and then return to a normal pattern.

Much of these cycle changes are the result of accelerated depletion of oocytes, which leads to eventual cessation of ovulation. Follicle depletion is manifested by significant changes in levels of hormones, especially estrogen[11]. As ovarian estrogen production decreases there is increased pituitary gland production of follicle stimulating hormone (FSH) to stimulate the ovary to secrete estrogen. However, FSH levels can fluctuate from month to month and from woman to woman during the perimenopause, which limits the utility of FSH as a predictor[12]. Elevated FSH levels cannot be used to predict when

menopause will begin. In general, menstrual cycle changes prior to menopause are marked by elevated FSH levels, decreased levels of inhibin and normal levels of luteinizing hormone (LH)[13]. Estradiol levels usually remain in the normal range until follicular growth and development cease. Estrogen levels have even been reported to increase before menopause[14]. Fluctuations of estrogen can become extreme during the perimenopause with wide variations in time and level. In a landmark longitudinal study, Santoro and co-workers[14] found that perimenopausal women tended to display a relatively hyperestrogenic state but also an inadequate progestogenic milieu. Menstrual cycle shortening with an accelerated follicular phase in ovulatory cycles alternates sporadically with anovulation. This results in perimenopausal women being more likely to suffer from anovulatory bleeding and puts such patients at increased risk for endometrial hyperplasia. Other medical conditions, some of which also predispose to anovulatory dysfunctional bleeding, are more likely to have their onset in midlife women. These include obesity, diabetes, thyroid disorders and hypertension.

The most urgent issue in clinical management is the exclusion of carcinoma or endometrial hyperplasia. The other component of clinical management is accurate assessment of the cause of the abnormal bleeding so that the most efficacious therapy can be instituted. The decision about whether the magnitude of abnormality in fact requires therapy, or can be simply managed with patient reassurance, is a complex clinical judgement. 'Symptomatic' bleeding in perimenopausal women is inextricably bound up in their fear that such bleeding is a sign that something is seriously wrong. Many such patients, if they can be assured that serious pathology (cancer or endometrial hyperplasia) is excluded, will often accept the inconveniences and quality of life issues that their degree of bleeding produces. It is often the fear of what the bleeding may signify that causes women to seek medical attention in the first place.

Diagnostic approachs to abnormal bleeding

It is clear that a perimenopausal patient with abnormal uterine bleeding needs evaluation. The vast majority will have dysfunctional uterine bleeding in association with episodes of anovulation that can best be managed hormonally or expectantly with reassurance. The value of an approach to distinguish such patients from those with organic pathological conditions in a safe, painless, convenient manner is obvious.

Initially, curettage was the gold standard. First described in 1843[15], its performance in the hospital became the most common operation performed in women worldwide. As early as the 1950s, a review of 6907 curettage procedures[16] found that the technique missed endometrial lesions in 10% of cases. Of these, 80% were polyps. A study of curettage before hysterectomy[17] found that in 16% of specimens less than one-quarter of the cavity was curetted, in 60% less than half of the cavity was curetted, and in 84% less than three-quarters of the endometrial cavity was effectively curetted.

In the 1970s, vacuum-suction curettage devices allowed sampling without anesthesia in an office setting. The most popular was the Vabra (Berkely Medevices, Berkely, CA) aspirator. This was found to be 86% accurate in diagnosing cancer[18]. Subsequently, cheaper, smaller, less painful plastic catheters with their own internal pistons to generate suction became popular. One of these, the Pipelle (Unimar, Wilton, CT) device, was found to have similar efficacy but better patient acceptance when compared with the Vabra[19].

Rodriguez and associates[20] carried out a pathological study of 25 hysterectomy specimens. The percentage of endometrial surface sampled by the Pipelle device was 4% versus 41% for the Vabra aspirator.

In one widely publicized study[21] the Pipelle had a 97.5% sensitivity to detect endometrial cancer in 40 patients undergoing hysterectomy. The shortcoming of that study was that the diagnosis of malignancy was known before the performance of the specimen collection.

In another study[22] Pipelle aspiration biopsy was performed in 135 premenopausal patients before curettage. Thirteen patients (10%) had different histological results on Pipelle biopsy as compared with curettage. It is interesting that only five of these patients had polyps, of which Pipelle sampling missed three. In total, 18 patients had hyperplasia, of which Pipelle sampling missed the diagnosis in seven (39%), thus underscoring the often focal nature of that pathological process.

Finally, in yet another study[23] Guido and colleagues also studied the Pipelle biopsy in patients with known carcinoma undergoing hysterectomy. Among 65 patients Pipelle biopsy provided tissue adequate for analysis in 63 (97%). Malignancy was detected in only 54 patients (83%). Of the 11 with false-negative results, five (8%) had disease confined to endometrial polyps and three (5%) had tumor localized to < 5% of the surface area. The surface area of the endometrial involvement in that study was ≤ 5% of the cavity in three of 65 (5%); 5–25% of the cavity in 12 of 65 (18%), of which the Pipelle missed four; 26–50% of the cavity in 20 of 65 (31%), of which the Pipelle missed four; and > 50% of the cavity in 30 of 65 patients (46%), of which the Pipelle missed none. These results provide great insight about the way endometrial carcinoma can be distributed over the endometrial surface or confined to a polyp. Because tumors localized in a polyp or a small area of endometrium may go undetected, the authors in that study concluded that the 'Pipelle is excellent for detecting global processes in the endometrium'.

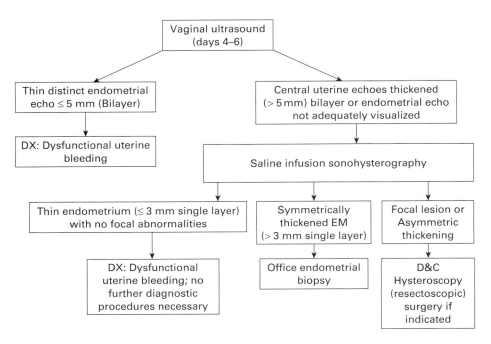

Figure 1 Flow chart for perimenopausal patients with abnormal uterine bleeding. DX, diagnosis; EM, endometrium; D&C, dilatation and curettage

From these data it seems that undirected sampling, whether through curettage or various types of suction aspiration, will often be fraught with error, especially in cases in which the abnormality is not global but focal (polyps, focal hyperplasia, or carcinoma involving small areas of the uterine cavity).

Hysteroscopy provides direct visualization of the endometrial cavity. Hysteroscopy with directed biopsy has been shown to be superior to curettage[24], although this procedure requires specialized equipment and is very operator dependent. It often requires ambulatory surgery centers and general anesthesia, or when it is performed as an office procedure with local or no anesthesia, it can potentially result in significant patient discomfort.

Transvaginal ultrasonography has been explored as an inexpensive, non-invasive, convenient way to indirectly visualize the endometrial cavity. It has been used most extensively in postmenopausal patients with abnormal bleeding. It has been shown effectively to exclude a lack of significant abnormality when the endometrial echo was ≤ 4 to 5 mm[25,26]. Premenopausal women have also been evaluated with transvaginal ultrasonography to exclude endometrial abnormalities when abnormal bleeding was present[27]. The addition of saline infusion sonohysterography can reliably distinguish perimenopausal patients with dysfunctional abnormal bleeding (no anatomic abnormality) from those with globally thickened endometria or those with focal abnormalities[28]. A clinical algorithm was proposed and studied in perimenopausal women with abnormal bleeding using unenhanced transvaginal ultrasonography, followed by saline infusion sonohysterography for selected patients, and then either no endometrial sampling, undirected endometrial sampling, or visually directed endometrial sampling, depending on whether the ultrasonographically based triage revealed no anatomic abnormality, globally thickened endometrium, or focal abnormalities, respectively[6] (Figure 1).

In that study 280 patients (65%) displayed a thin, distinct, symmetric endometrial echo

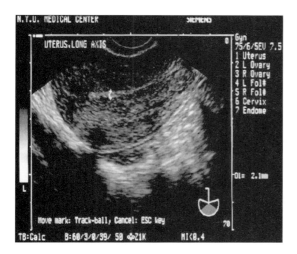

Figure 2 Endovaginal ultrasonography on day 6, revealing a thin distinct endometrial echo measuring 2.1 mm (calipers) on this long-axis view. This picture excludes significant abnormality and is compatible with proliferative endometrial tissue on histological examination

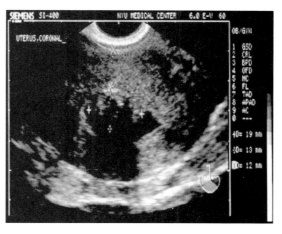

Figure 4 Coronal view of patient depicted in Figure 3. There is an anterior wall midline submucous myoma measuring 1.9 × 1.3 cm. The endometrium surrounding the fluid instillation is thin, indicative of proliferative histology

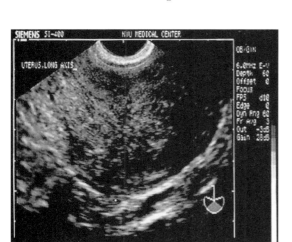

Figure 3 Long-axis view of the uterus in a patient with menometrorrhagia. A distinct endometrial echo is not well visualized. This is an indication for saline infusion sonohysterography

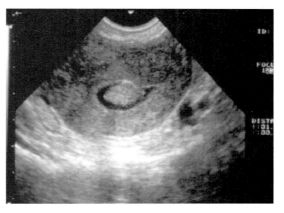

Figure 5 Long-axis view of the uterus in a patient with abnormal uterine bleeding. There is a polyp protruding from the anterior wall approximately half way to the fundus. It measures 1.5 × 0.9 cm (calipers). The echogenic endometrium that overlies the fluid lining the remainder of the cavity is thin and in the early proliferative stage, compatible with a lack of significant abnormality

of ≤ 5 mm on days 4–6, and dysfunctional uterine bleeding was diagnosed (Figure 2). A total of 153 (35%) had saline infusion sonohysterography. Of these procedures, 44 (29%) were performed because of the inability to characterize and measure the endometrium adequately (Figures 3 and 4) and 109 (71%) were performed for an endometrial measurement of ≥ 5 mm. Of those patients, 61 then had both anterior and posterior endometrial thickness that was symmetric and < 3 mm, compatible with dysfunctional uterine bleeding. Fifty-eight patients (13%) had focal polypoid masses (Figure 5) that were removed

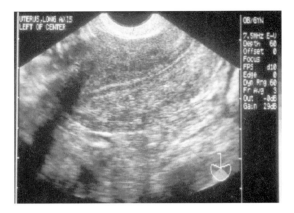

Figure 6 Long-axis view of the uterus in a perimenopausal patient with irregular bleeding. The seemingly normal endometrial echo is taken to the left of center. This is a two-dimensional snapshot. This one frozen image may not be representative of the entire endometrial cavity

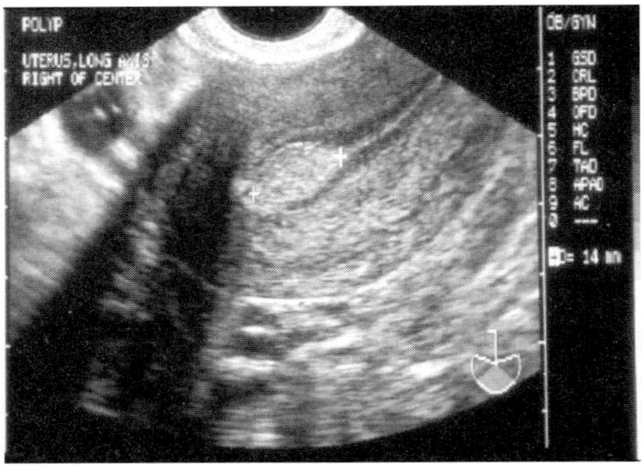

Figure 7 Same patient as in Figure 6. This long-axis view to the right of center clearly shows an endometrial polyp not appreciated in the scanning plane shown in Figure 6

hysteroscopically and confirmed pathologically. Twenty-two patients (5%) had submucous myomas, although 148 patients (34%) had clinical and ultrasonographic evidence of fibroids. Ten patients had single-layer measurements of the endometrium by saline infusion sonohysterography of > 3 mm (range 3–9 mm). Of these, histological type was proliferative endometrium in five and hyperplastic endometrium in five. Saline infusion sonohysterography was technically inadequate in two patients who then underwent hysteroscopy with curettage. Undirected office biopsy alone without imaging potentially would have missed the diagnosis of focal lesions such as polyps, submucous myomas and focal hyperplasia in up to 80 patients (18%).

A reliable assessment with ultrasonography requires that the endometrial echo be homogeneous, surrounded by an intact hypoechoic junctional zone, and that the operator constantly remember that the endometrial cavity is a three-dimensional structure. This may account for why Dijkhuzien and co-workers[27] had four cases that supposedly measured < 10 mm (some as little as 2 mm) and yet at hysteroscopy displayed polyps. Such cases underscore the importance of the three-dimensional character of the endometrial cavity and the occasional propensity of the ultrasonographic operator to obtain a limited number of two-dimensional views and assume that these represent the entire endometrial cavity. Any single 'frozen' ultrasonographic image is nothing more than a two-dimensional snapshot, and failure to recreate three-dimensional anatomy meticulously will result in error (Figures 6 and 7).

Another potential pitfall of saline infusion sonohysterography is the irregular topographic surface of the endometrial cavity as it proliferates. The sonohysterography procedure is very time sensitive and should be performed as the bleeding episode ends when the endometrial thickness can be expected to be at its thinnest. Delaying the procedure can result in the development of a sizeable amount of endometrial tissue that can be mistaken for small polyps or focal hyperplasia, leading to inappropriate further interventions. Such a sonographic appearance is reminiscent of 'moguls' on a ski slope (Figure 8).

Therapy

The therapy of abnormal uterine bleeding could certainly be the subject of an entire chapter of its own. Appropriate therapy,

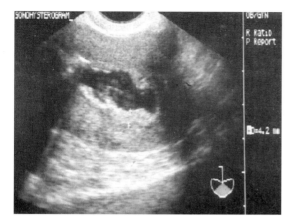

Figure 8 Long-axis view of a patient with abnormal perimenopausal bleeding. This is 17 days since the last bleeding episode ended. The irregular topography referred to as endometrial 'moguls' is not uncommon and is not distinguishable sonographically from small polyps or areas of focal hyperplasia

however, begins with accurate diagnosis of the source of the bleeding. With few exceptions, invasive cancer mandates hysterectomy and surgical staging. The majority of women with complex hyperplasia with cytological atypia (carcinoma *in situ*), especially when reproductive function is no longer an issue, will be best treated with simple hysterectomy, although the use of progestins to treat all forms of hyperplasia has been employed. Leiomyomata, depending on their size, location, amount of bleeding, and patient preference, can be handled by hysterectomy, myomectomy (by a variety of routes) or expectant management. Recently uterine artery embolization has been postulated and utilized for therapy. Other techniques in the future may include therapeutic ultrasound to ablate such lesions. Endometrial polyps can be removed hysteroscopically. Their prevalence is high. In perimenopausal women with any break in bleeding cyclicity the incidence was reported to be 13%[6]. The incidence of malignancy in the polyps of such patients is low, ranging from 0.5 to 1.5%[29]. Attempts to utilize color Doppler ultrasound to predict which polyps are malignant or even hyperplastic have not proved to be successful[30].

Dysfunctional uterine bleeding, as discussed above, can be equated with anovulatory estrogen withdrawal bleeding when anatomic causes have been excluded. Unopposed estrogen stimulates proliferation of the endometrium and the cumulative effect of constant estrogen stimulation, depending on dose and duration, is positively correlated with the risk of developing endometrial neoplasia. In ovulating women, luteal progesterone secretion obviates this risk by inducing a decidual change within the endometrium, halting the estrogen-induced proliferation, and converting it irreversibly to secretory endometrium. In the absence of pregnancy, the corpus luteum spontaneously regresses, ending inevitably in menstruation and the universal shedding of the endometrium. The loss of endometrial tissue reduces the likelihood of progression from proliferation to neoplasia. The goal of medical therapy for dysfunctional uterine bleeding should be to replace the hormonal control missing in anovulatory women, that is, the effect of luteal progesterone.

One therapeutic approach is administration of oral progestins for 10–14 days every 1–2 months to induce withdrawal bleeding. In this strategy, the effect of the continuous estrogen action on the endometrium is counteracted by a pharmacological course of progestin to simulate the effect of progesterone in the luteal phase. This treatment, however, does not alter gonadotropin secretion, does not prevent the occasional spontaneous ovulation and, therefore, does not provide contraception. Additionally, non-ovulatory bleeding episodes are still common, as the endogenous estrogen production continues unabated.

Traditional hormone replacement therapy (HRT) used in menopause, that is, conjugated estrogen with added progestin, has sometimes been prescribed for perimenopausal women. Such regimens are not enough to suppress ovarian activity[31] and may occasionally provide excessive amounts of estrogen that can cause side-effects. Owing to the lack of suppression of ovarian activity with standard-dose

HRT regimens, alternative methods of contraception are still necessary. In using traditional HRT in such patients, the cyclic progestins in these regimens may be helpful in inducing endometrial sloughing, but adding pharmacological doses of estrogen to an already estrogenized endometrium may intensify the problem. This causes more, rather than less, endometrial proliferation, worsening the amount and irregularity of vaginal bleeding.

In perimenopausal women, the most successful strategy for treating dysfunctonal uterine bleeding is the use of combined oral contraceptives. This is a very cost-effective medical intervention, providing excellent cycle control and significantly reducing the amount of menstrual blood loss, dysmenorrhea and the likelihood of progression from proliferation to neoplastic endometrium. The constant progestin in the pill suppresses gonadotropin secretion and reduces endogenous estrogen production, so the endometrium is exposed only to the exogenously administered hormone. Also, this regimen prevents ovulation and provides contraception, something lacking in the other medical treatments.

The American College of Obstetricians and Gynecologists recommends that such medical therapies be offered prior to surgical intervention for dysfunctional uterine bleeding, mainly because of reduced cost and risks, unless they are otherwise contraindicated[5]. Surgical therapy is indicated for women with excessive anovulatory bleeding in whom medical management has failed, assuming that they have completed their childbearing. Appropriate goals for medical therapy include avoidance of anemia, reduction of excessively heavy bleeding and improved predictability of bleeding.

A surgical alternative to hysterectomy is ablation of the endometrium, and this can be performed by a variety of techniques both approved and some still investigational. These include Yag laser, endometrial resection, rollerball or rollerbarrel coagulation, or thermal injury by heat or freezing. Studies have compared cost and surgical outcomes between endometrial resection or ablation and hysterectomy. Hysteroscopic ablation is more cost-effective than hysterectomy and results in less morbidity and shorter recovery periods[32]. This must be balanced against the fact that one-third of women who undergo endometrial ablation will undergo hysterectomy within the following 5 years[33].

Summary

Abnormal uterine bleeding in midlife women is common. The clinician needs to exclude uterine malignancy or hyperplasia but furthermore needs to diagnose the etiology of the bleeding in order to tailor various therapeutic options for each individual patient. This is best accomplished with a thorough understanding of the physiological and pathological conditions that result in such bleeding as well as the various diagnostic and therapeutic modalities currently available.

References

1. Shwayder JM. Contemporary management of abnormal uterine bleeding. *Obstet Gynecol Clin* 2000;27:219–34
2. Nesse R. Abnormal vaginal bleeding in perimenopausal women. *Am Fam Physician* 1989;40:185–9
3. World Health Oganization. Report of a WHO Scientific Group. *Research on the Menopause in the 1990's*. WHO Technical Report Series 866. Geneva: WHO, 1996
4. SEER cancer statistics review, 1973–1996 (serial online). Available at http://ww-seer./imsnci.nih.gov/Publications/CSR1973 1996
5. American College of Obstetricians and Gynecologists. *Management of Anovulatory Bleeding*. Practice Bulletin, Washington: ACOG, 2000;14:961–8

6. Goldstein SR, Zelster I, Horan CK, Snyder JR, Schwartz LB. Ultrasonography-based triage for perimenopausal patients with abnormal uterine bleeding. *Am J Obstet Gynecol* 1997;177:102–8

7. McKinlay SM, Brambilla PJ, Posner JG. The normal menopause transition. *Maturitas* 1992;14:103–15

8. Lenton EA, Landgren BM, Sexton L, Harper R. Normal variation in the length of the follicular phase of the menstrual cycle: effect of chronological age. *Br J Obstet Gynaecol* 1984;91:681–4

9. Treolar AE, Bonton RE, Behn BG, *et al*. Variation of the human menstrual cycle through reproductive life. *Int J Fertil* 1967;12:77–127

10. Sherman BM, Korenman SG. Hormonal characteristics of the human menstrual cycle throughout reproductive life. *J Clin Invest* 1975;55:699–706

11. Richardson SJ, Senikas V, Nelson JF. Follicular depletion during the menopausal transition: evidence for accelerated loss and ultimate exhaustion. *J Clin Endocrinol Metab* 1987;65:1231–7

12. Stellato RK, Crawford SL, McKinlay SM, Longcope CL. Can follicle-stimulating hormone be used to define menopausal status? *Endocr Pract* 1998;4:137–41

13. Burger HG, Dudley EC, Hopper JL, *et al*. The endocrinology of the menopausal transition: a cross-sectional study of a population-based sample. *J Clin Endocrinol Metab* 1995;80:3537–45

14. Santoro N, Brown JR, Adel T, Skurnick JG. Characterization of reproductive hormonal dynamics in the perimenopause. *J Clin Endocrinol Metab* 1996;81:1495–501

15. Ricci JV. Gynaecologic surgery and instruments of the nineteenth century prior to the antiseptic age. In *The Development of Gynaecological Surgery and Instruments*. Philadelphia: Blakiston, 1949:326–8

16. Word B, Gravlee LC, Widemon GL. The fallacy of simple uterine curettage. *Obstet Gynecol* 1958;12:642–5

17. Stoch RJ, Kanbour A. Prehysterectomy curettage. *Obstet Gynecol* 1975;45:537–41

18. Vuopala S. Diagnostic accuracy and clinical applicability of cytological and histological methods for investigating endometrial carcinoma. *Acta Obstet Gynecol Scand Suppl* 1997;70:1

19. Kaunitz AM, Masciello AS, Ostrowsky M, Rovvira EZ. Comparison of endometrial Pipelle and Vabra aspirator. *J Reprod Med* 1988;33:427–31

20. Rodriguez MJ, Platt LD, Medearis AL, Lacarra M, Lobo RA. The use of transvaginal sonography for evaluation of postmenopausal size and morphology. *Am J Obstet Gynecol* 1988;159:810–14

21. Stoval TG, Photopulos GJ, Poston WM, Ling FW, Sandles LG. Pipelle endometrial sampling in patients with known endometrial cancer. *Obstet Gynecol* 1991;77:954–6

22. Goldchmit R, Katz A, Blickstein I, Caspi B, Dgani R. The accuracy of endometrial Pipelle sampling with and without sonographic measurement of endometrial thickness. *Obstet Gynecol* 1993;82:727–30

23. Guido RS, Kanbour A, Ruhn M, Christopherson WA. Pipelle endometrial sampling sensitivity in the detection of endometrial cancer. *J Reprod Med* 1995;40:553–5

24. Gimpelson R, Roppold H. A comparative study between panoramic hysteroscopy with directed biopsies and dilatation and curettage. *Am J Obstet Gynecol* 1988;158:489–94

25. Goldstein SR, Nachtigall M, Snyder JR, Nactigall L. Endometrial assessment by vaginal ultrasonography before endometrial sampling in patients with postmenopausal bleeding. *Am J Obstet Gynecol* 1990;163:119–23

26. Langer RD, Pierce JJ, O'Hanlan KA, *et al*. Transvaginal ultrasonography compared with endometrial biopsy for the detection of endometrial disease. *N Engl J Med* 1997;337:1792–8

27. Dijkhuizen FPHLJ, Brolmann HAM, Potters AE, Bongers MY, Heinz AP. The accuracy of transvaginal ultrasonography in the diagnosis of endometrial abnormalities. *Obstet Gynecol* 1996;87:345–9

28. Goldstein SR. Use of ultrasonohysterography for triage of perimenopausal patients with unexplained uterine bleeding. *Am J Obstet Gynecol* 1994;170:565–70

29. Anastasiadis PG, Koutlaki NG, Skaphida PG, Galazios GC, Tsikouras PN, Liberis VA. Endometrial polyps: prevalence, detection, and malignant potential in women with abnormal uterine bleeding. *Eur J Gynaecol Oncol* 2000;21:180–3

30. Goldstein SR, Monteagudo A, Popiolek D, Mayberry P, Timor-Tritsch I. Evaluation of endometrial polyps. *Am J Obstet Gynecol* 2002;186:669–74

31. Glasier A, Gebbie A. Contraception for the older woman. *Baillière's Clin Obstet Gynecol* 1996;10:121–38

32. Brooks PG, Clouse J, Morris LS. Hysterectomy vs. resectoscopic endometrial ablation for the control of abnormal uterine bleeding. A cost-comparative study. *J Reprod Med* 1994;39:755–60

33. Gannon MJ, Holt EM, Fairbank J, *et al*. A randomized trial comparing endometrial

resection and abdominal hysterectomy for the treatment of menorrhagia. *Br Med J* 1991;303: 1362–4

34. Indman PD. Hysteroscopic treatment of menorrhagia associated with uterine leiomyomas. *Obstet Gynecol* 1993;81:716–20

35. Towbin NA, Gviazda IM, March CM. Office hysteroscopy versus transvaginal ultrasonography in the evaluation of patients with excessive uterine bleeding. *Am J Obstet Gynecol* 1996;174:1678–82

Screening for major malignancies in the perimenopausal woman

9

V. A. Givens and F. W. Ling

Introduction

In the year 2002, an estimated 1 284 900 new cases of invasive cancer will be diagnosed in the USA and approximately 553 400 Americans will die as a result of cancer. For women, the incidence will be roughly 647 400 with a death toll of 267 300[1]. Remarkably, these numbers do not include either basal or squamous cell cancer of the skin, which are expected to account for more than a million new cases during the same time period. Women between the ages of 40 and 59 have a 1/11 chance of developing some type of invasive cancer. In comparison, females from birth to age 39 have only a 1/51 chance of being diagnosed with cancer. Cancer mortality rates for women from the year 1999 are shown according to age in Table 1. As this table illustrates, knowledge about cancer screening becomes exceedingly important for practitioners involved in primary and preventive care of women as they approach menopause.

There are four major considerations when choosing cancer screening protocols. First, the test must be effective in finding cancer in asymptomatic patients. Next, the test must detect the cancer early enough to allow treatment and a subsequent reduction in morbidity and mortality. The risk of performing the screening procedure must be overshadowed by the benefit of finding and treating the cancer. Furthermore, the test should prove to be practical and feasible in an office setting. Once a test meets all these criteria, it may be employed as a screening test.

Guidelines concerning the use of screening tests are generally established by medical organizations or government agencies. Examples of groups who offer such guidelines are the American College of Obstetricians and Gynecologists (ACOG), the American Academy of Family Practice (AAFP), the American Medical Association (AMA), the

Table 1 Mortality from cancer in women according to age group in 1999 – the leading five sites are presented for each age group. The approximate percentages of the total number of deaths for each specific age group are shown. From reference 1

| | Age (years) | | | | | |
| | 20–39 | | 40–59 | | 60–79 | |
	n	%	n	%	n	%
All sites	5747		46 747		131 972	
Breast	1426	24.8	11 525	25	17 773	13.5
Cervix	519	9	—	—	—	—
Leukemia	494	8.6	—	—	—	—
Lung and bronchus	432	7.5	10 182	22	38 260	29
Nervous system/brain	384	6.7	—	—	—	—
Colon and rectum	—	—	3 571	7.5	12 940	10
Ovary	—	—	2 964	6	7 100	5
Pancreas	—	—	1 860	4	7 747	6
Others	2492	43.4	16 645	35.6	48 152	36.5

Table 2 Guide to the US Preventive Service Task Force ratings for screening tests[13]

A   There is good evidence to support the recommendation that the condition be specifically considered in a periodic health examination

B   There is fair evidence to support the recommendation that the condition be specifically considered in a periodic health examination

C   There is insufficient evidence to recommend for or against the inclusion of the condition in a periodic health examination, but recommendations may be made on other grounds

D   There is fair evidence to support the recommendation that the condition be excluded from consideration in a periodic health examination

E   There is good evidence to support the recommendation that the condition be excluded from consideration in a periodic health examination

American Cancer Society (ACS), the American Gastroenterological Association (AGA) and the US Preventive Services Task Force (USPSTF). Since the recommendations for each group vary slightly, it is up to each practitioner to individualize the guidelines for a specific patient. To date, the recommendations of the USPSTF and the Canadian Task Force on the Periodic Health Examination (CTFPHC) provide the most scientific, least biased framework for evaluating which preventive health measures should be included in the routine care of individuals. The USPSTF assigns each screening test a letter (A–E) based on the strength of the evidence in support of the intervention (Table 2). These letters will be included in the tables of recommendations for each screening test.

Regardless of the group of guidelines used, the overall goal for using screening tests is to reduce morbidity and mortality by identifying disease in asymptomatic patients. This chapter will focus on perimenopausal women at low risk. Recommendations for this population are typically given for ages 45–65 years. Patients may be screened more frequently based on individual risk factors, which will also be listed along with accepted screening modalities.

Breast cancer

Despite enhanced awareness about breast cancer, it remains the overall leading non-cutaneous site of cancer among women in the Western world, and it accounts for the largest number of cancer deaths in women aged 20–59. The often quoted 1 in 8 risk for a woman developing breast cancer is based on a lifetime risk for a 90 year old. In the year 2001 alone, an estimated 192 000 cases of breast cancer were newly diagnosed, and there were approximately 40 200 deaths[2]. Unfortunately, the incidence is expected to rise to 203 500 cases in 2002 (not including an additional 54 300 cases of breast carcinoma *in situ*). On the other hand, a slightly decreased mortality rate is expected[1]. In addition to improvements in the treatment of breast cancer, the decrease in mortality may be attributed to identifying more cases at an early stage through screening tests. Five-year survival is much improved if breast cancer is diagnosed while still localized (97%), and is progressively poorer for regional (77%) and distant (22%) disease[3]. The three most commonly recommended screening modalities for detecting breast cancer are mammography, clinical breast examination and self-breast examination. Numerous clinical trials have evaluated these screening tests. Based on the results of these clinical trials, medical organizations have developed recommendations for screening the general population. It is widely accepted that mammography is the most effective screening test for the early detection of breast cancer; nonetheless, most protocols include a combination of self-breast examination and clinical breast examination. These subjective examinations are included to identify potential masses that

Table 3 Recommendations for use of screening by mammography

AAFP[14]	every 1–2 years for ages 50–69; counsel women aged 40–49 about potential risks and benefits
ACOG[15]	every 1–2 years for ages 40 to 49; annually for ages 50 and above
ACS[16]	annually after age 40
AMA[17]	every 1–2 years for ages 40–49; annually for ages 50 and above
CTFPHC[18]	every 1–2 years for ages 50–59
USPSTF[19]	every 1–2 years for ages 50–69 ('A' recommendation); for women aged 40–49, there is conflicting evidence of fair to good quality regarding clinical benefit ('C' recommendation); women aged 70 and older should be screened based on other grounds such as life expectancy and patient preference

AAFP, American Academy of Family Practice; ACOG, American College of Obstetricians and Gynecologists; ACS, American Cancer Society; AMA, American Medical Association; CTFPHC, Canadian Task Force on the Periodic Health Examination; USPSTF, United States Preventive Services Task Force

Table 4 Recommendations for use of clinical breast examinations

AAFP[14]	every 1–2 years for ages 50–69; counsel women aged 40–49 about potential risks and benefits
ACOG[15]	annually with yearly examination (does not specify ages)
ACS[16]	ages 20–39, every 3 years; age 40 and above, annually prior to mammogram so that clinically evident lesions may be marked for diagnostic mammography. (Both tests should be performed within a short period of time)
AMA[17]	every 1–2 years for ages 40–49; annually for ages 50 and older
CTFPHC[18]	annually for ages 50–69
USPSTF[19]	every 1–2 years for ages 50–69 is optional; insufficient evidence to recommend for or against using this alone ('C' recommendation)

See Table 3 for definition of terms

were not detected on mammography owing to test limitations, rapid tumor growth or human error (Tables 3–5).

Patients who are considered at higher risk for developing cancer may be screened more

Table 5 Recommendations for use of self-breast examinations

AAFP[14]	no recommendations
ACOG[15]	no recommendations
ACS[16]	monthly beginning at age 20
AMA[17]	no recommendations
CTFPHC[18]	no recommendations
USPSTF[19]	there is insufficient evidence to recommend for or against teaching self-breast examination in the periodic health examination ('C' recommendation)

See Table 3 for definition of terms

frequently at the discretion of their health-care provider. High-risk factors generally include menarche at younger than 14 years, nulliparity, completing a first live birth after 30 years of age and menopause at age 55 or older[4–7]. The Gail model for assessing risk of developing breast cancer also includes increasing age, race, number of prior breast biopsies, a diagnosis of atypical hyperplasia and the number of first-degree relatives with breast cancer[8]. In addition, familial cancer syndromes (*BRCA-1* and *BRCA-2*) increase the risk of being diagnosed with breast cancer. It is beyond the scope of this chapter to address them in detail (see Chapter 12 on reduction of breast cancer risk).

Cervical cancer

An estimated 12 900 cases of cervical cancer were diagnosed in the USA in 2001 and 4400 women died as a result[2]. These numbers are similar to the expected incidence and mortality in 2002[1]. Approximately half of all patients diagnosed with cervical cancer have not had a Papanicolaou (PAP) test performed within the previous 5 years. The PAP test has accomplished the goals of a good screening test. It recognizes asymptomatic, preinvasive disease and subsequently allows for earlier treatment and, ultimately, better outcomes. Since the introduction of PAP screening, mortality rates from cervical cancer have decreased by more than 80%.

Table 6 Papanicolaou (PAP) test guidelines

AAFP[14]	at least every 3 years beginning with sexual intercourse for women with a cervix
ACOG[15]	annually beginning at age 18 or when sexually active; after three or more tests with normal results, may be performed less frequently on physician's advice
ACS[16]	annually beginning at age 18 or when sexually active; after two or three normal results, continue at discretion of the physician
AMA[17]	annually beginning at age 18 or when sexually active; after three or more normal annual PAP tests, may be performed less frequently at discretion of the physician
CTFPHC[18]	annually beginning at age 18 or when sexually active; after two normal results, test every 3 years to age 69
USPSTF[19]	test all women who have ever had sexual intercourse and who have a cervix ('A' recommendation); frequency of testing should be at least every 3 years ('B' recommendation); may stop regular testing after age 65 if results have been consistently normal ('C' recommendation)

See Table 3 for definition of terms

Recommendations for screening of generalized populations with PAP tests are outlined in Table 6. The Medicare definition of a high-risk population includes one or more of the following: age 16 or younger at first sexual intercourse, multiple sexual partners (five or more), a history of sexually transmitted disease (including human immunodeficiency virus (HIV) infection) or fewer than three normal PAP tests in the previous 7 years. While not included in the Medicare definition of high risk, tobacco use, low socioeconomic status and human papilloma virus infection are other commonly cited risk factors.

Whereas ACOG, ACS, AMA and CTFPHC all recommend screening beginning at age 18 or with initiation of sexual activity, the AAFP and USPSTF do not suggest beginning testing at any specific age. Likewise, the frequency of testing is debated among the organizations. Most agree that less frequent screening for low-risk patients may be undertaken following two or three cytologically normal, satisfactory PAP tests. It has been shown that performing PAP tests every 1–2 years, as compared with every 3 years, improves screening effectiveness by less than 5%[9].

Colorectal cancer

In the year 2002, an estimated 77 900 cases of cancer of the colon, rectum or anus will be diagnosed in women in the USA[1]. This is a 10% increase in incidence from the year

2001[2]. Approximately 29 100 deaths are expected, making it the third most lethal cancer in perimenopausal women[1]. Survival rates for colorectal cancer are dependent on the stage of diagnosis. The commonly reported 5-year survival rate is 91% if the disease is diagnosed while still localized; however, only 66% of patients will survive 5 years if the disease is regionally spread. Even more impressive is that the overall 5-year survival decreases to only 9% with distant metastasis. With widespread use of screening procedures, more cancers are diagnosed early which leads to a markedly improved survival.

Screening procedures that are commonly used for the detection of colorectal cancer include digital rectal examination (DRE), fecal occult blood test (FOBT), double contrast barium enema (DCBE), sigmoidoscopy and colonoscopy. These screening procedures have two goals. The first is diagnosis of colorectal cancer in its early stages in order to improve survival. The second goal is removal of adenomatous polyps subsequently preventing progression to invasive cancer. The recommendations presented here are for low-risk patients (Tables 7–10). Risk factors for colorectal cancer are listed in Table 11. The consensus regarding testing high-risk patients is that screening should begin at an earlier age, and with an increased frequency. The exact age at which to begin screening and the frequency at which to evaluate these patients still varies according to organization. Referral

Table 7 Guidelines for screening with digital rectal examinations

AAFP[14]	no published standards for low-risk patients
ACOG[15]	> 50 years old, should accompany pelvic examination annually and with each colonoscopy or sigmoidoscopy
ACS[16]	> 50 years old, every 5 years with sigmoidoscopy orDCBE; every 10 years with colonoscopy
AMA[17]	no recommendations
AGA[14]	no recommendations
CTFPHC[18]	insufficient evidence to recommend use
USPSTF[21]	insufficient evidence to recommend use ('C' recommendation)

DCBE, double contrast barium enema; see Table 3 for definition of other terms

Table 8 Guidelines for screening with the fecal occult blood test

AAFP[14]	no published standards for low-risk patients
ACOG[15]	annually after age 50
ACS[16]	annually after age 50
AMA[17]	annually after age 50
AGA[14]	beginning at age 59 (frequency not specified)
CTFPHC[18]	insufficient evidence to recommend use
USPSTF[21]	annually after age 50 ('B' recommendation)

see Table 3 for definition of terms

to a gastroenterologist for management of high-risk patients is quite appropriate.

Ovarian cancer

Despite advances in treatment regimens and attempts at developing screening protocols, ovarian cancer remains the deadliest of all the gynecological malignancies. Likewise, it is the fourth leading cause of cancer death in perimenopausal women. This is mainly attributable to the lack of symptoms experienced by the affected patient until the disease has spread widely. The lifetime incidence of developing ovarian cancer is 1 in 70. In the year 2002, 23 300 new cases of ovarian cancer will be diagnosed in perimenopausal women, and 13 900 patients will die as a result of the disease[1]. These deaths account for more than

Table 9 Screening with the double contrast barium enema

AAFP[14]	no published standards for low-risk patients
ACOG[15]	no recommendations
ACS[16]	after age 50, may use this with DRE every 5–10 years
AMA[17]	no recommendations
AGA[14]	beginning at age 59, may use this every 5–10 years
CTFPHC[18]	no recommendations
USPSTF[21]	insufficient evidence to recommend use ('C' recommendation)

DRE, digital rectal examination; see Table 3 for definition of other terms

Table 10 Screening using either flexible sigmoidoscopy or colonoscopy

AAFP[14]	no published standards for low-risk patients
ACOG[15]	after age 50, sigmoidoscopy every 5 years with yearly FOBT or colonoscopy every 10 years with yearly FOBT; in addition, DRE should be performed with each colonoscopy or sigmoidoscopy
ACS[16]	after age 50, sigmoidoscopy with FOBT and DRE every 5 years or colonoscopy and DRE every 10 years
AMA[17]	after age 50, sigmoidoscopy every 3–5 years
AGA[14]	beginning at age 59, sigmoidoscopy every 5 years or colonoscopy every 10 years
CTFPHC[18]	insufficient evidence to recommend use of either modality
USPSTF[21]	after age 50, may use sigmoidoscopy with FOBT ('B' recommendation); the task force did not specify an interval

FOBT, fecal occult blood test; DRE, digital rectal examination; see Table 3 for definition of other terms

those occurring from cervical, endometrial, vulvar and vaginal malignancies combined.

Not unlike other types of malignancy, ovarian cancer has a much better prognosis when diagnosed in its early stages. The 5-year survival rate for a properly staged patient with local disease is 80% or better. The survival drops to approximately 30% for regional metastasis, and further decreases to only 5% if the disease is widely metastatic at presentation. Regrettably, most ovarian cancers are metastatic to some degree when diagnosed. This is why

Table 11 Established risk factors for developing colorectal cancer

Personal history of colorectal cancer
History of cancer or polyps in a first-degree relative before age 60
History of cancer or polyps in two or more first-degree relatives at any age
Adenomatous polyps
Familial polyposis
Hereditary non-polyposis colorectal cancer
Ulcerative colitis

Table 12 Symptoms suggestive of lung cancer

Persistent cough
Chest pain, often aggravated by deep breathing
Hoarseness
Weight loss and loss of appetite
Bloody or rust-colored sputum
Shortness of breath
Fever without known reason
Recurrent lung infections
New-onset wheezing

the importance of searching for an adequate screening test cannot be overstated.

Potential screening tests for ovarian cancer include bimanual examination, transvaginal ultrasonography and serum tumor marker testing (CA-125 in particular). The sensitivity of bimanual examination is unknown; however, it is assumed to be low, based on the location of the ovary and differences between examiners. Most ovarian cancers found using only bimanual examination are in advanced stages.

Ultrasound screening seems feasible for early detection of ovarian cancer, but its use is limited by its high rate of false-positive results. These false-positive results often lead to much more invasive diagnostic modalities such as laparoscopy or laparotomy which significantly increase health-care costs and potentially have serious complications. Based on the available studies, it has been estimated that ultrasound screening of 100 000 women over age 45 would detect only 40 cases of ovarian cancer, with 5 398 false-positive results, and more than 160 complications from laparoscopy[10]. These studies are generally limited by small sample sizes, limited follow-up and lack of randomization. Further studies using this modality of screening are warranted.

Biochemical markers are currently used to monitor patients who are known to have certain types of ovarian cancer. CA-125 levels are often present with epithelial ovarian cancers; however, they are elevated in only about half of all cases. They may also be elevated in other conditions including endometriosis, uterine leiomyomata, benign ovarian cysts, neoplasms other than those of ovarian orgin and pelvic inflammatory disease. More research using a combination of serum screening and ultrasound, particularly with color flow Doppler, may be useful in the future.

Considering the low sensitivity of serum tumor markers and the low specificity of ultrasound, most organizations align themselves with the USPSTF, which states that routine screening for ovarian cancer by ultrasound, the measurement of serum tumor markers, or pelvic examination is not recommended ('D' recommendation). In addition, there is insufficient evidence to recommend for or against the screening of asymptomatic women at increased risk of developing ovarian cancer ('C' recommendation)[9].

Unfortunately, 95% of all ovarian cancers occur in women without risk factors. Since women at high risk account for 5–10% of all cases, they should be identified and potentially offered screening on a research protocol. Risk factors for developing ovarian cancer include the familial cancer syndromes (BRCA-1, BRCA-2, HPNCC syndrome, and Lynch II syndrome), family history of ovarian cancer (no specific syndrome), nulliparity, age > 35 at first pregnancy and the use of ovulation induction medications.

Lung cancer

In the USA, more than 90% of lung cancer cases are related to cigarette smoking[11]. Unfortunately, cancer of the lung and bronchus is second only to breast cancer in the number of expected deaths in perimenopausal women in the year 2002. During this year, 79 200 new cases are expected to be diagnosed, and approximately 65 700 deaths will be credited to lung cancer[1]. The high mortality to case ratio is attributable to the dismal prognosis of most lung cancers. The overall 5-year survival rate for all stages is only 5–14%[11]. Both sputum cytology and serial chest X-rays have been proposed as screening tests for lung cancer. However, the results of eight prospective studies conducted over the last 40 years (including over 39 000 total patients) have failed to show any reduction in the mortality associated with lung cancer. This is true even for high-risk populations. Currently, new studies are being

performed using low-dose helical computed tomography. In time, we may have a feasible screening modality for lung cancer.

Currently, the best recommendation for all patients regarding lung cancer is to avoid exposure to cancer-inducing agents. In addition to the carcinogens in cigarette smoke, working around asbestos, radon, uranium, arsenic and vinyl chloride has also been associated with the development of lung cancer. If a patient continues to smoke or to be exposed to second-hand smoke or other carcinogens, she should be advised to report any symptoms immediately (Table 12). The USPSTF states that routine screening of asymptomatic patients for lung cancer is not recommended ('D' rating)[12].

References

1. Jemal A, Thomas A, Murray T, Thun M. Cancer statistics, 2002. *CA Cancer J Clin* 2002;52:23–47
2. Greenlee R, Hill-Harmon M, Murray T, Thun M. Cancer statistics, 2001. *CA Cancer J Clin* 2001;51:15–36
3. Eyre HJ, Smith RA, Mettlin CJ. *Cancer Screening and Early Detection*, 5th edn. Hamilton, Ontario: B.C. Decker Inc., 2000
4. Kelsey JL, Berkowitz GS. Breast cancer epidemiology. *Cancer Res* 1988;48:5615–23
5. Kelsey JL, Gammon MD. Epidemiology of breast cancer. *Epidemiol Rev* 1990;12:228–40
6. Kelsey JL, Gammon MD. The epidemiology of breast cancer. *CA Cancer J Clin* 1991;41:146–65
7. Kelsey JL, Gammon MD, John EM. Reproductive factors and breast cancer. *Epidemiol Rev* 1993;15:36–47
8. Gail M, Brinton L, Byar D, *et al.* Projecting individualized probabilities of developing breast cancer for white females who are being examined annually. *J Natl Cancer Inst* 1989;81: 1879–86
9. Campbell S, Bhan V, Royston J, *et al.* Screening for early ovarian cancer. *Lancet* 1998;1:710–11
10. USPSTF. Screening for ovarian cancer. In Fisher M, Eckart C, eds. *Guide to Clinical Preventive Services*, 2nd edn. Baltimore: Williams and Wilkins, 1996:159–66
11. Frame PS. Routine screening for lung cancer? Maybe someday, but not yet. *J Am Med Assoc* 2000;284:1980–3
12. USPSTF. Screening for lung cancer. In Fisher M, Eckart C, eds. *Guide to Clinical Preventive*

Services, 2nd edn. Baltimore: Williams and Wilkins, 1996:135–9
13. USPSTF. Task force ratings. In Fisher M, Eckart C, eds. *Guide to Clinical Preventive Services*. Baltimore: Williams & Wilkins, 1996:387
14. Zoorob R, Anderson R, Cefalu C, Sidani M. Cancer screening guidelines. *Am Fam Physician* 2001;63:1101–12
15. American College of Obstetricians and Gynecologists. *Routine Cancer Screening*. ACOG Committee Opinion No. 247. Washington, DC: ACOG, 2000
16. Smith RA, Cokkinides V, von Eschenbach AC, *et al.* American Cancer Society Guidelines for the early detection of cancer. *CA Cancer J Clin* 2002;52:8–22
17. American Medical Association. *Cancer Screening Guidelines*. Available at http://www.ama-assn.org
18. Examination CTFotPH. *Canadian Guide to Clinical Preventive Health Care*. Ottawa: Canada Communication Group, 1994
19. USPSTF. Screening for breast cancer. In Fisher M, Eckart C, eds. *Guide to Clinical Preventive Services*, 2nd edn. Baltimore: Williams and Wilkins, 1996:73–87
20. USPSTF. Screening for cervical cancer. In Fisher M, Eckart C, eds. *Guide to Clinical Preventive Services*, 2nd edn. Baltimore: Williams and Wilkins, 1996:105–17
21. USPSTF. Screening for colorectal cancer. In Fisher M, Eckart C, eds. *Guide to Clinical Preventive Services*, 2nd edn. Baltimore: Williams and Wilkins, 1996:89–103

Uterine disease in midlife women 10

R. L. Barbieri

In this chapter, the diagnosis and treatment of benign diseases of the uterus, including leiomyomata uteri (myomas), adenomyosis, endometrial polyps and endometrial hyperplasia, are discussed.

Leiomyomata uteri

Leiomyomata uteri, also known as fibroids or uterine myomas, are benign smooth muscle tumors of the uterus. Myomas are the most common pelvic tumor in women, occurring in approximately 20% of women of reproductive age. In some series, up to 70% of hysterectomy procedures are performed to treat myomas.

Etiology

An important and exciting advance in gynecology is the identification of a small number of genes that are mutated in uterine myomas, but not in normal myometrial cells. The clinical implications of this discovery have been described in detail in other publications[1-3]. Myomas are monoclonal tumors, suggesting that they arise from a somatic mutation in a single precursor myocyte. Approximately 45% of myomas are cytogenetically abnormal, with the most frequently affected chromosomes being 1, 6, 7, 12 and 14. The most frequently reported cytogenetic abnormalities in myomas are: del(7)(q22q32), t(12;14) (q15,q23–24); t(1;2)(p36,p24) and rearrangements involving 6p21[4]. Mutations in chromosomes 1 and 7 probably result in the loss of function of a tumor suppressor gene. Translocation between chromosomes 12 and 14 results in the activation of a growth-promoting gene, *HMGI-C*, which is active in

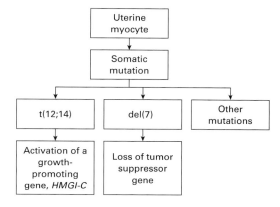

Figure 1 The somatic mutation theory of uterine leiomyomata states that each myoma is a monoclonal tumor derived from a single precursor myocyte that underwent a critical somatic mutation. In women with multiple myomas, each tumor arises from an independent somatic mutation. Current evidence indicates that a small number of critical genes are the targets of the mutations that cause myomas. The t(12;14) translocation, the most common somatic mutation observed in myomas, appears to activate a growth-promoting gene, *HMGI-C*. The del(7) and 1q mutations appear to cause the deletion of a tumor suppressor gene. These tumor suppressor genes have not yet been identified

fetal life, and normally quiescent in adult life[5] (Figure 1).

Of all the mutations causing myomas, the molecular biology of the t(12;14) translocation is best understood. The t(12;14) translocation appears to activate a member of the high-mobility group of genes, *HMGI-C*. *HMGI-C* is a DNA architectural factor that influences DNA conformation, regulating the effects of transcription factors on gene expression. HMGI-C protein binds to the minor groove of AT-rich DNA through the AT hook domain. HMGI-C is phosphorylated by p34/cdc2-like kinases. The phosphorylation

Table 1 Uterine leiomyomata with t(12;14) translocations are larger than leiomyomata with del(7) mutations. Original table using data from reference 6

Karyotype abnormality	Mean diameter of largest myoma removed from uterus (cm)	Calculated myoma volume (cm³)
t(12;14)	10.6	421
del(7)	4.1	48

state of the protein influences its affinity for DNA. In fetal life, *HMGI-C* is actively expressed in many tissues. In adult life, *HMGI-C* expression is repressed in normal cells. The t(12;14) translocation in a uterine myocyte causes the induction of *HMGI-C* expression, which in turn causes the clonal expansion of the myocyte into a uterine fibroid. Mutations in chromosome 12q15, at the locus of the *HMGI-C* gene, are also associated with human lipomas, angiomyxomas, breast fibroadenomas, pulmonary chondroid hamartomas, endometrial polyps and salivary gland adenomas[4].

Interestingly, the size of uterine myomas appears to be related, in part, to the chromosomal abnormality. In one study, myomas with a del(7) chromosomal abnormality had a mean diameter of 4.1 cm. In contrast, myomas with a t(12;14) translocation had a mean diameter of 10.6 cm (Table 1). In addition, uterine leiomyomata with all metaphases demonstrating abnormal chromosome rearrangements are typically larger than myomas with normal metaphases or myomas with a mixed pattern of normal and some abnormal metaphases[6].

Uterine myomas are primarily caused by a mutation in a progenitor myocyte. However, hormonal factors, such as estrogen and progesterone, probably control the frequency of critical mutations and the rate of progression of the tumors. Uterine myomas appear to be more sensitive to estrogen than normal myocytes from the same uterus[7]. Because estrogen is a growth factor/stimulator of uterine myocyte growth and function, increased sensitivity to estrogen could account for the propensity of uterine myomas to grow in midlife women.

Anatomic and histological classification

Myomas are classified as submucosal (beneath the endometrium), intramural (centered in the muscular wall of the uterus) or subserosal (beneath the uterine serosa). Both submucosal and subserosal tumors may become pedunculated. Myomas overproduce collagen, which contributes to their firmness and pale coloration. Most myomas are hyalinized. About 10% of myomas contain significant areas of hemorrhage. Most myomas have fewer than five mitoses per ten high-power fields. Leiomyosarcomas typically have more than ten mitoses per ten high-power fields. In this cancer many of the cells demonstrate features of cellular atypia.

Epidemiology

The epidemiology of uterine myomas has been studied in depth in a cohort of 95 061 premenopausal nurses 25–44 years of age with intact uteri[8]. During the 4 years of the study, 4181 new cases of myoma were diagnosed by ultrasound or surgery. The observed incidence rate increased with advancing age and was greatest in African-American women (Figure 2). The peak incidence of myomas was in the age range of 40–44 years. In the age range of 25–29 years, the incidence of myomas was three and six new cases per 1000 woman-years for Caucasian and African-American women, respectively. In the age range of 40–44 years, the incidence was approximately 15 and 35 new cases per 1000 woman-years for Caucasian and African-American women, respectively. Age-standardized incidence rates by race were 8.9 new cases per 1000 woman-years for

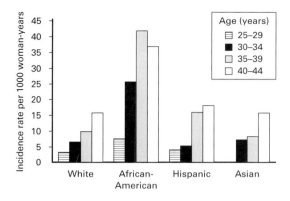

Figure 2 Incidence rates of uterine leiomyomata confirmed by ultrasound or hysterectomy according to age and race among premenopausal women in the Nurses' Health Study II, 1989–1993. From reference 8

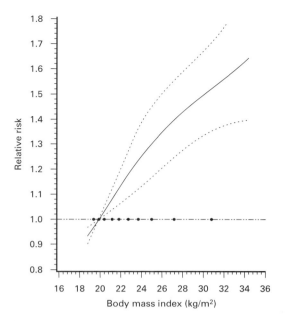

Figure 3 Non-parametric regression curve of the relation between body mass index (BMI) and the risk of uterine leiomyomata confirmed by ultrasound or hysterectomy among premenopausal women in the Nurses' Health Study II, 1989–1993. The dotted lines represent 95% confidence limits. The black circles represent the deciles of the distribution of BMI in this population. From reference 9

Caucasian women and 30.6 new cases per 1000 woman-years for African-American women. Hispanic and Asian women had incidence rates similar to those observed in Caucasian non-Hispanic women: 11 and 8 new cases per 1000 woman-years, respectively. The increased incidence of uterine myomas observed in black women persisted after controlling for the effects of age, body mass index (BMI), reproductive history, socioeconomic class and smoking. Genetic and hormonal factors may account for the observed effect of race on the incidence of myomas. Interestingly, a number of recent reports indicate that African-American women may have higher circulating estrogen levels than Caucasian women.

BMI is a modifiable factor that was associated with an increased risk of myomas (Figure 3). A BMI of 28–30 kg/m^2 increased the risk of myomas[9] by 1.36 compared with a referent BMI of 20–22 kg/m^2. Significant weight gain after age 18 increased the risk of developing myomas. Increased BMI may be associated with increased estrogen production and increased bioavailability of growth factors such as insulin-like growth factor-I (IGF-I). The incidence of other estrogen- and growth factor-dependent diseases, such as breast and endometrial cancer, is also increased in women with increased BMI.

Parity decreases the risk of uterine myomas (Table 2). Parous women had a 0.67 risk of developing myomas compared with nulliparous women[10]. The protective effect of parity decreased as the number of years since the last birth increased. Early menarche was associated with an increased risk of developing uterine leiomyomata. Women with menarche before age 10 had a 1.51 risk of developing myomas compared with women with menarche after age 12. The use of oral contraceptives did not influence the risk of developing myomas.

Treatment of uterine myomas

Women with uterine myomas most often present for treatment for the following symptoms and signs: a newly diagnosed pelvic mass; abnormal uterine bleeding; pelvic pain or pressure; and infertility.

Table 2 Influence of parity on the risk of uterine leiomyomata. From reference 10

	Person-years	Number of incident cases	Age-adjusted relative risk and 95% CI	Multivariate relative risk and 95% CI
Nulliparous	90 548	949	1.00	1.00
Parous	232 517	2026	0.67 (0.62–0.72)	0.67 (0.61–0.74)

CI, confidence interval

The newly diagnosed pelvic mass

A common clinical problem is the discovery of a new pelvic mass in a midlife woman. A new pelvic mass may be caused by tumors of the uterus, ovary or bowel. A pelvic ultrasound examination has high sensitivity and specificity for diagnosing ovarian and uterine tumors and should be performed in all women with a newly diagnosed pelvic mass. Uterine myomas and uterine leiomyosarcomas may be difficult to differentiate using physical examination and a pelvic sonogram. In one study of 1332 women undergoing hysterectomy for a newly diagnosed pelvic mass thought to be a uterine myoma, 0.23% of the women were diagnosed as having a uterine leiomyosarcoma, endometrial stromal sarcoma or a mixed mesodermal tumor[11]. In another study of 1432 women planning to have a hysterectomy for presumed benign uterine disease, 0.49% had leiomyosarcoma diagnosed at the time of surgery[12]. Many uterine leiomyosarcomas grow rapidly, whereas most uterine myomas grow very slowly. A woman with a newly diagnosed pelvic mass thought to be a uterine myoma should be examined every 6 months for 2 years to help determine whether the tumor is growing slowly or rapidly. Rapidly growing uterine tumors typically require surgical treatment. In many women with uterine leiomyosarcomas, constitutional symptoms such as weight loss, fever and night sweats are present.

Abnormal uterine bleeding

In a midlife woman with a myoma, abnormal uterine bleeding can be exacerbated both by hormonal abnormalities and by the uterine tumor. Perimenopause is associated with a hormonal pattern of relative estrogen excess and progesterone deficiency. The estrogen excess–progesterone deficiency pattern can contribute to menorrhagia by altering the normal pattern of endometrial growth–differentiation and shedding. In addition, the estrogen excess–progesterone deficiency pattern may stimulate an increase in the growth and cellular activity of uterine myomas. Uterine myomas induce abnormal blood vessel growth and function in the endometrium adjacent to the myoma[13]. A protein related to the transforming growth factor-β superfamily, endometrial bleeding associated factor (ebaf), has been reported to be significantly overexpressed in the endometrium of women with menorrhagia[14]. It is possible that ebaf disrupts the ability of the endometrial blood vessels to seal themselves during menstruation.

Women with menorrhagia and a pelvic mass thought to be a uterine myoma by physical examination and pelvic sonogram may need both an endometrial biopsy and a diagnostic hysteroscopy. The endometrial biopsy is highly effective at detecting endometrial cancer and hyperplasia. Diagnostic hysteroscopy, which can be performed in the office setting without anesthesia using a 3-mm flexible hysteroscope, is highly effective at detecting submucosal myomas. An alternative is to perform saline infusion hysterosonography. If a submucosal myoma is identified in a woman with menorrhagia, the lesion should be removed by operative hysteroscopy. In one study, 75% of women with menorrhagia and submucosal myomas treated with operative hysteroscopy showed resolution of their menorrhagia[15]. For women with menorrhagia and intramural or submucosal myomas, treatment options include: pharmacological therapy, endometrial ablation, placement of an intrauterine progestin-releasing system, myomectomy and hysterectomy.

Pharmacological treatment

For women with menorrhagia and a uterine myoma, pharmacological treatment can be tried prior to surgical intervention. In women with primary menorrhagia, ibuprofen at a dose of 1200 mg daily has been reported to reduce menstrual blood loss from 146 ml to 110 ml. However, in women with menorrhagia and uterine myomas, this dose of ibuprofen did not reduce menstrual blood loss[16]. A large-scale clinical trial of oral contraceptives to treat menorrhagia in women with uterine myomas has not been reported. Many clinicians believe that oral contraceptive treatment can be effective in reducing menorrhagia in a subgroup of women with myomas and menorrhagia. A few women with menorrhagia and myomas may have an increase in myoma volume when treated with oral contraceptives[17].

Mifepristone, also called the 'abortion pill' or RU-486, has been demonstrated to reduce myoma volume by approximately 50% and, at appropriate doses, to induce amenorrhea. An advantage of antiprogestin therapy is that endogenous estradiol levels are not suppressed into the menopausal range. Mifepristone does not cause as much bone loss as long-term gonadotropin releasing hormone (GnRH) agonist treatment[18]. It is likely that a number of antiprogestins will be developed to treat myomas in the next 10 years.

Endometrial ablation

Endometrial ablation, with either hysteroscopic endometrial resection or rollerball coagulation[19], or with a balloon thermal technique, is effective in reducing menorrhagia in women with enlarged uteri due to leiomyomata uteri. In most series about 75% of the treated women have a clinically acceptable reduction in menstrual bleeding[20]. The main complication associated with hysteroscopic endometrial ablation is fluid overload, which can result in hyponatremia and death. Myoma coagulation or myolysis is associated with a reduction in the size of the uterine myoma, but not with marked improvement in menorrhagia.

Intrauterine progestin-releasing system

The levonorgestrel-releasing intrauterine system (Mirena®) may be effective in the treatment of menorrhagia associated with uterine myomas. In one phase II study, the device was fitted in 12 women with menorrhagia and uterine myomas. Follow-up at 6 months revealed that the majority of women had reduced menstrual bleeding. However, one woman failed to respond and had surgical treatment[21].

Myomectomy and hysterectomy

Some women with menorrhagia and intramural or subserosal myomas will need myomectomy or hysterectomy to treat their menorrhagia. In the USA, the surgical treatment of myomas is dominated by the hysterectomy procedure. Approximately nine hysterectomy procedures for myomas are performed for every one myomectomy procedure. Many surgeons believe that myomectomy is associated with a higher rate of morbidity than is hysterectomy, despite recent evidence indicating that surgical morbidity is very low for both procedures. In one study, myomectomy was associated with a lower risk of bladder and bowel injury but with greater blood loss than hysterectomy[22]. For women with submucous myoma, hysteroscopic myomectomy is very effective in reducing menorrhagia[23]. In one study of 285 women with 5 years of follow-up, hysteroscopic resection of submuocus myomas resulted in reduction in menstrual bleeding in 90% of women. Numerous clinical trials have reported that, in women with menorrhagia, anemia and myomas, treatment with a GnRH agonist analog prior to myomectomy or hysterectomy can increase blood volume and decrease the chance of receiving a blood transfusion during the perioperative interval[24].

Many women with menorrhagia and myomas will choose hysterectomy as their preferred treatment. In this clinical setting, hysterectomy is associated with an improvement in quality of life in over 90% of women[25]. Vaginal hysterectomy is associated with more rapid recovery than abdominal hysterectomy. A challenge for the gynecological surgeon is to maximize the number of vaginal hysterectomy procedures that can be safely performed in this clinical situation. Every gynecological surgeon has an upper limit to the size of uterus that he or she is comfortable removing by a vaginal approach. GnRH agonists have been demonstrated to decrease the size of myomas, so that more vaginal hysterectomy procedures can be performed.

In one study, 50 premenopausal women with myomas and a uterine size in the range of 14–18 gestational weeks were randomized to group A (no preoperative hormone treatment followed by hysterectomy) or group B (8 weeks of preoperative GnRH agonist treatment (depot leuprolide acetate 3.75 mg intramuscularly every 4 weeks for 8 weeks) followed by hysterectomy[26]. Women in group B, the GnRH agonist-treated group, had an increase in hemoglobin concentration from 11 g/dl to 12 g/dl ($p < 0.05$) and a decrease in uterine size from 1090 cm to 723 cm ($p < 0.05$). Women in group B, the GnRH agonist-treated group, were more likely to have a vaginal hysterectomy than women in group A: 76% vs. 16%, respectively. The cost of the preoperative GnRH agonist treatment was offset by the reduced hospitalization of the women who had a vaginal hysterectomy. This study suggests that, in women with myomas for whom a hysterectomy is planned, preoperative treatment with a GnRH agonist for 8–12 weeks will increase the frequency of successful vaginal hysterectomy.

Uterine artery embolization

Uterine artery (UA) embolization is a percutaneous angiography procedure performed by an interventional radiologist. The femoral artery is catheterized and a small (5-Fr) angiographic catheter is threaded into the UA. After ensuring that the catheter is placed in the proper anatomic location, polyvinyl alcohol particles are delivered into the UA. Owing to the relatively high blood flow to uterine myomas, the particles are carried preferentially into the circulation arcade of the myomas. Some radiologists leave a gelatin sponge or a steel coil in the UA at the end of the procedure as an additional uterine occlusive modality.

UA embolization was first utilized in the treatment of severe postpartum hemorrhage, where surgical intervention had failed or was contraindicated. UA embolization has been reported to be successful in the treatment of a variety of severe bleeding problems such as uterine arteriovenous malformations, gestational trophoblastic disease, pelvic trauma and cervical ectopic pregnancy. Recently, many centers have reported the successful use of UA embolization in the treatment of menorrhagia associated with uterine myomas. In one report, 16 women with myomas and menorrhagia were treated with UA embolization. During short-term follow-up, it was observed that 11 women had significant improvement in their menorrhagia, three had partial resolution and two required surgical intervention[27]. To date, no randomized clinical trial has been reported that compares UA embolization with another method of treating menorrhagia due to myomas. In addition, most reports of UA embolization do not provide information concerning long-term follow-up of the treated women.

Current contraindications to UA embolization include: a desire for future fertility; a co-existing malignancy; allergy to contrast media; active pelvic inflammatory disease; and current use of GnRH agonists. GnRH agonists decrease the caliber of the UA and make it difficult to catheterize the vessel[28]. Another problem with UA embolization is that no uterine tissue is obtained for pathological evaluation. There are many case reports of women with pelvic masses thought to be myomas, which were treated without

Table 3 Impact of uterine leiomyomata on reported infertility. From reference 10

History of infertility	Person-years	Number of incident cases	Age-adjusted relative risk and 95% CI	Multivariate relative risk and 95% CI
Yes	54 191	658	1.26 (1.15–1.37)	1.28 (1.17–1.41)
No	271 926	2348	1.00	1.00

CI, confidence interval

surgery and were later demonstrated to be leiomyosarcomas or bowel cancer. Management of pelvic masses thought to be fibroids without a pathological diagnosis is likely to result in an occasional misdiagnosis.

A major problem with UA embolization is that post-procedure pain can be severe. Many centers use regional anesthesia and patient-controlled narcotic analgesia to treat post-procedure pain but many women require hospitalization. Post-embolization syndrome occurs in approximately 15% of treated women and is characterized by prolonged post-procedure pain, leukocytosis and gastrointestinal symptoms (nausea and vomiting). Although not common, ovarian failure has occurred post-procedure. Death has also been reported following the procedure in association with severe necrosis and infection of the uterus and fatal sepsis[29].

Pelvic pain and pressure

Some women with uterine myomas report pelvic pain and pelvic pressure. Studies using microtransducer recordings of uterine pressure have reported that some women with uterine myomas have increased uterine muscle contractility that can be associated with the sensation of cramping, pressure and pain. In some women with myomas, the uterus has expanded to fill the entire anterior cul-de-sac, resulting in pressure on the bladder that is perceived as urinary symptoms such as urinary frequency.

Infertility

Uterine myomas probably cause a modest degree of subfertility. In one study, the presence of uterine myomas was associated with a relative risk of infertility of 1.28 compared with the lack of myomas[10] (Table 3). Some studies have suggested that, of the three types of myoma, the submucosal myomas are the most likely to contribute to infertility[30]. Many women with uterine myomas are more than 35 years of age. After 35 years, ovarian aging and a depleted oocyte pool may contribute to the infertility problem.

Adenomyosis

Adenomyosis is the presence of endometrial glands and stroma in the myometrium, at least 2 mm below the endomyometrial junction. Adenomyosis is commonly associated with the clinical triad of menorrhagia, dysmenorrhea and a slightly enlarged, 'boggy' uterus on physical examination. The pathogenesis of adenomyosis is poorly characterized, but many authorities believe that invasion of the basoendometrium into the myometrium gives rise to foci of adenomyosis. Uterine trauma at the time of delivery, increased uterine pressure or chronic endometritis may increase the likelihood that the basoendometrium will invade into the myometrium. Alternatively, preliminary evidence suggests that some adenomyosis lesions may be monoclonal and that a mutation in a precursor cell may give rise to adenomyosis lesions. Numerous epidemiological studies have reported that adenomyosis is not observed before menarche and is seldom diagnosed more than 5 years after the menopause. Parous women appear to be at increased risk for adenomyosis. This contrasts with endometriosis, which is much more common in nulliparous women.

The diagnosis of adenomyosis is typically made on a hysterectomy specimen. There are no widely accepted, non-surgical methods for diagnosing adenomyosis. The normal endomyometrial junction is irregular, with endometrial glands and stroma dipping into the myometrium for a variable distance. Many pathologists define adenomyosis as the presence of endometrial glands and stoma in the myometrium more than 2–3 mm below the endomyometrial junction. The sensitivity of the pathological diagnosis of adenomyosis is highly correlated with the number of myometrial sections processed for analysis from the hysterectomy specimen. In one study of 200 consecutive hysterectomy specimens, the investigators reported that processing three myometrial sections resulted in 62 women being identified with adenomyosis, but that processing six myometrial sections resulted in 123 women being identified with adenomyosis. Autopsy studies of midlife women revealed that approximately 50% of the women had adenomyosis. Some studies report that the deeper the myometrial invasion, the more severe the reported menorrhagia and dysmenorrhea. Most uteri of patients with adenomyosis weigh between 100 and 200 g and are seldom larger than a gestational size of 12 weeks.

Adenomyosis can be diagnosed only by histological analysis of myometrial sections. Adenomyosis may be present when the clinical triad of menorrhagia, dysmenorrhea and a slightly enlarged uterus is observed in a parous woman with a pelvic ultrasound examination that demonstrates no uterine myomas. Most women with adenomyosis are between 35 and 50 years of age when the diagnosis is made. Investigators have attempted to develop imaging studies to diagnose adenomyosis; but most have reported that the sensitivity and specificity of the imaging studies are not adequate to recommend their use as a definitive test modality. For example, in one study of transvaginal ultrasound, the sensitivity and specificity for the diagnosis of adenomyosis was 86% and 50%, respectively[31]. In one study of magnetic resonance imaging to diagnose adenomyosis, the sensitivity and specificity of the test was 20% and 100%, respectively.

Hysterectomy is the only treatment that is clearly effective in the treatment of adenomyosis. Preliminary studies have reported that hormonal therapies effective in the treatment of uterine myomas (GnRH agonist analogs) may also be effective in the treatment of adenomyosis[32,33].

Endometrial polyps

An endometrial polyp is a benign tumor consisting of surface endometrium lining three sides of the tumor, fibrous stroma and thick-walled, centrally positioned blood vessels. Preliminary reports indicate that clonal rearrangement of chromosome 6p21 is observed in some mesenchymal (stroma) cells in endometrial polyps[34]. One possible explanation of this finding is that an endometrial polyp begins when a stromal cell undergoes a rearrangement in chromosome 6p21, resulting in an abnormal signal to grow. The stromal elements proliferate and bring the endometrial glands along as 'innocent bystanders'. Of interest, 6p21 is the locus of a gene HMGI-Y, which is related to the gene HMGI-C, which causes some cases of uterine myomas.

Polyps are typically suspected in women with abnormal uterine bleeding. Polyps are usually diagnosed by pelvic ultrasonography, office hysteroscopy, saline infusion hysterosonography or hysterosalpingogram. In menopausal women taking estrogen–progestin hormone replacement therapy who have abnormal uterine bleeding, polyps are present in up to 20% of cases. Office hysteroscopy can efficiently diagnose endometrial polyps in this clinical setting[35]. Tamoxifen treatment is associated with the development of endometrial polyps.

Endometrial hyperplasia

Endometrial hyperplasia is usually due to the dual hormone defect of excess estrogen and inadequate progesterone. In the Postmenopausal Estrogen and Progestin Interventions

(PEPI) trial, women in one treatment arm were treated with estrogen alone (conjugated equine estrogen 0.625 mg daily), without concomitant progestin treatment. In this estrogen-only group, 20% of the women developed endometrial hyperplasia in the first year of therapy[36]. Mutations in a tumor suppressor gene, *PTEN*, are observed in about 50% of women with endometrial hyperplasia[37]. In the endometrium, loss of *PTEN* activity increases both cell growth and estrogen sensitivity.

Women with excess estrogen and decreased progesterone production include: perimenopausal women, women with polycystic ovary syndrome and obese oligo-ovulatory women. These women are at the highest risk for endometrial hyperplasia and should undergo endometrial sampling if abnormal uterine bleeding is present. In addition, women using unopposed estrogen should have an endometrial biopsy. In women with abnormal uterine bleeding and a low risk of endometrial hyperplasia, transvaginal ultrasound may be an effective screening modality. In one study, no endometrial cancers were detected if the endometrial stripe was < 4 mm in diameter[38]. If the endometrium is > 4 mm in diameter, an endometrial biopsy should be obtained.

Simple hyperplasia without atypia progresses to malignancy in less than 2% of cases. Complex hyperplasia with cytological atypia can progress to cancer in about 20% of cases. All cases of complex hyperplasia with cytological atypia require treatment. Hormone treatment with high-dose progestin is effective in most cases. Typical regimens include megesterol acetate, 40 mg two to four times daily[39]. An endometrial biopsy should be performed after 12 weeks of treatment to assess the efficacy of the regimen. Once regression of the endometrial hyperplasia is demonstrated, the progestin dose can be reduced. Hysterectomy is an option for women who have completed their family.

Summary

Diseases of the uterus are among the most common medical problems of midlife women. Genetic mutations and hormonal changes (high estrogen–low progesterone) influence the risk of developing uterine diseases in midlife. Advances in genetics and hormone treatment (selective estrogen receptor modulators, antiprogestins) offer hope that, in the near future, uterine diseases in midlife women will be preventable.

References

1. Barbieri RL, Andersen J. Uterine leiomyomas: the somatic mutation theory. *Semin Reprod Endocrinol* 1992;10:301–9
2. Barbieri RL. Ambulatory management of uterine leiomyomata. *Clin Obstet Gynecol* 1999;42:196–205
3. American College of Obstetricians and Gynecologists. *Precis: Gynecology. Disorders of the Uterus*. Washington, DC: ACOG, 1998:34–9
4. Ligon AH, Morton CC. Genetics of uterine leiomyomata. *Genes Chromosomes Cancer* 2000;28:235–45
5. Schoenmakers EF, Wanschura S, Mols R, Cullerdiek J, Ven den Berghe H, Van de Ven WJ. Recurrent rearrangements in the high mobility group protein gene, HMGI-C in benign mesenchymal tumors. *Nature Genet* 1995;10:436–44
6. Rein MS, Powell WL, Walters FC, *et al.* Cytogenetic abnormalities in uterine myomas are associated with myoma size. *Mol Hum Reprod* 1998;4:83–6
7. Andersen J, DyReyes VM, Barbieri RL, Coachman DM, Miksicek RJ. Leiomyoma primary cultures have elevated transcriptional response to estrogen compared with autologous myometrial cultures. *J Soc Gynecol Invest* 1995;2:542–51
8. Marshall LM, Spiegelman D, Barbieri RL, *et al.* Variation in the incidence of uterine leiomyomata among premenopausal women by age and race. *Obstet Gynecol* 1997;90:967–73
9. Marshall LM, Spiegelman D, Goldman MB, *et al.* Risk of uterine leiomyomata among premenopausal women in relation to body size and cigarette smoking. *Epidemiology* 1998;9:511–17

10. Marshall LM, Spiegelman D, Goldman MB, *et al.* A prospective study of reproductive factors and oral contraceptive use in relation to the risk of uterine leiomyomata. *Fertil Steril* 1998;70:432–9

11. Parker WH, Fu YS, Berek JS. Uterine sarcoma in patients operated on for presumed leiomyoma and rapidly growing leiomyoma. *Obstet Gynecol* 1994;83:414–18

12. Leibsohn S, d'Ablaing G, Mishell DR, Schlaerth JB. Leiomyosarcoma in a series of hysterectomies performed for presumed uterine leiomyomas. *Am J Obstet Gynecol* 1990;162: 968–74

13. Stewart EA, Nowak RA. Leiomyoma related bleeding: a classic hypothesis updated for the molecular era. *Hum Reprod Update* 1996;2: 295–306

14. Kothapalli R, Buyiksal I, Wu SQ, Chegini N, Tabibzadeh S. Detection of ebaf, a novel human gene of the transforming growth factor beta superfamily – association of gene expression with endometrial bleeding. *J Clin Invest* 1997;99:2342–50

15. Derman SG, Rehnstrom J, Neuwirth RS. The long-term effectiveness of hysteroscopic treatment of menorrhagia and leiomyomas. *Obstet Gynecol* 1991;77:591–4

16. Makarainen L, Ylikorkala O. Primary and myoma-associated menorrhagia: role of prostaglandins and effects of ibuprofen. *Br J Obstet Gynaecol* 1986;93:974–8

17. Barbieri RL. Reduction in the size of a uterine leiomyoma following discontinuation of an estrogen–progestin contraceptive. *Gynecol Obstet Invest* 1997;43:276–7

18. Murphy AA, Kettel LM, Morales AJ, Roberts VJ, Yen SS. Regression of uterine leiomyomata in response to the anti-progesterone RU-486. *J Clin Endocrinol Metab* 1993;76:513–17

19. Eskandar MA, Vilos GA, Aletebi FA, Tummon IS. Hysteroscopic endometrial ablation is an effective alternative to hysterectomy in women with menorrhagia and large uteri. *J Am Assoc Gynecol Laparosc* 2000;7:339–45

20. Vilos GA, Vilos EC, King JH. Experience with 800 hysteroscopic endometrial ablations. *J Am Assoc Gynecol Laparosc* 1996;4:33–8

21. Starczewski A, Iwanicki M. Intrauterine therapy with levonorgestrel releasing IUD of women with hypermenorrhea secondary to uterine fibroids. *Ginekol Polska* 2000;71:1221–5

22. Iverson RE, Chelmow D, Strohbehn K, Waldman L, Evantash EG. Relative morbidity of abdominal hysterectomy and myomectomy for management of uterine leiomyomas. *Obstet Gynecol* 1996;88:415–19

23. Emanuel MH, Wamsteker K, Hart AA, Metz G, Lammes FB. Long-term results of hysteroscopic myomectomy for abnormal uterine bleeding. *Obstet Gynecol* 1999;93:743–8

24. Candiani GB, Vercellini P, Fedele L, Arcaini L, Bianchi S. Use of goserelin depot for the treatment of menorrhagia and severe anemia in women with leiomyomata uteri. *Acta Obstet Gynecol Scand* 1990;69:413

25. Carlson KJ, Miller BA, Fowler FJ. The Maine women's health study. I: Outcomes of hysterectomy. *Obstet Gynecol* 1994;83:556

26. Stovall TG, Ling FW, Henry LC, Woodruff MR. A randomized trial evaluating leuprolide acetate before hysterectomy as treatment for leiomyomas. *Am J Obstet Gynecol* 1991;164:1420–3

27. Ravina JH, Herbreteau D, Ciraru-Vigneron N, *et al.* Arterial embolization to treat uterine myomata. *Lancet* 1995;346:671–2

28. Siskin GP, Stainken BF, Dowling K, Meo P, Ahn J, Dolen EG. Outpatient uterine artery embolization for symptomatic uterine fibroids: experience in 49 patients. *J Vasc Inter Radiol* 2000;11:305–11

29. Vashisht A, Studd J, Carey A, Burn P. Fatal septicemia after fibroid embolization. *Lancet* 1999;354:307–8

30. Farhi J, Ashkenazi J, Feldberg D, Dicker D, Orvieto R, Rafael Z. Effect of uterine leiomyomata on results of IVF treatment. *Hum Reprod* 1995;10:2576–8

31. Brosens JJ, de Souza NM, Barker FG, Paraschos T, Winston RM. Endovaginal ultrasonography in the diagnosis of adenomyosis uteri: identifying and predictive characteristics. *Br J Obstet Gynaecol* 1995;102:471–4

32. Silva PD, Perkins HE, Schauberger CW. Live birth after treatment of severe adenomyosis with a gonadotropin releasing hormone agonist. *Fertil Steril* 1994;61:171–2

33. Hirata JD, Moghissi KS, Ginsburg KA. Pregnancy after medical therapy of adenomyosis with a gonadotropin-releasing hormone agonist: a case report. *Fertil Steril* 1993; 59:444–5

34. Fletcher JA, Pinkus JL, Lage JM, Morton CC, Pinkus GS. Clonal 6p21 rearrangement is restricted to the mesenchymal component of an endometrial polyp. *Genes Chromosomes Cancer* 1992;5:260–3

35. Widrich R, Bradley LD, Mitchinson AR, Collins RL. Comparison of saline infusion sonography with office hysteroscopy for the evaluation of the endometrium. *Am J Obstet Gynecol* 1996;174:1327–34

36. The Writing Group for the PEPI Trial. Effects of hormone replacement therapy on endometrial

histology in postmenopausal women. *J Am Med Assoc* 1996;275:370–5

37. Mutter GL, Lin McFitzgerald JT, Kum JB, Baa KJP, Lees JA. Altered PTEN expression as a diagnostic marker for the earliest endometrial precancers. *J Natl Cancer Inst* 2000;92:924–31

38. Karlsson B, Gransberg S, Wikland M, *et al.* Transvaginal sonography of the endometrium

in women with postmenopausal bleeding. *Am J Obstet Gynecol* 1995;172:1488–94

39. Randall TC, Kurman RJ. Progestin treatment of atypical hyperplasia and well-differentiated carcinoma of the endometrium in women under age 40. *Obstet Gynecol* 1997;90:434–40

Creative use of oral contraceptives in the perimenopausal patient

11

P. J. Sulak

Introduction

Oral contraceptives (OCs) are underutilized in perimenopausal women. In fact, many women discontinue OCs in their thirties, when they or their spouse opt for sterilization. Unfortunately, this is the phase in a woman's reproductive life when OCs are often most beneficial. The fluctuating ovarian function seen in the perimenopause can last for several years and can begin in the mid- to late thirties in some patients. Declining quantity and quality of follicles, rising follicle stimulating hormone (FSH) levels, and fluctuating estrogen and progesterone levels can result in shortened menstrual cycles and/or menstrual irregularity[1]. A hyperestrogenic state, accompanied by a luteal phase progesterone decrease, is seen in many perimenopausal patients and can eventually result in heavy menses, anemia, hyperplasia and the growth of fibroids. Because OCs inhibit gonadotropin production and thus ovarian hormone production, they are the ideal method of management, not only for treatment of these common sequelae of declining ovarian function but, importantly, for prevention of these gynecological disorders. Prevention is preferable to treatment, because many of these conditions require diagnostic procedures and surgical intervention, with associated costs and morbidity.

Benefical effects of perimenopausal oral contraceptive use

The beneficial effects of perimenopausal OC use are so numerous that one could make a case for their recommendation as a primary preventive therapy (Table 1). Many women in their thirties to early fifties do not desire to use an intrauterine device or undergo sterilization and therefore need some other reliable form of contraception. OC use negates the need for these procedures. Importantly, women over the age of 40 can experience unintended pregnancy, often leading to elective abortion[2]. OCs also reduce the risk of ectopic pregnancy. By continuing OCs up until the menopause, permanent sterilization is unnecessary. Studies have shown that women who have had tubal ligations have a higher incidence of hysterectomy[3–5], and a significant percentage request tubal reversal[6]. Also, tubal ligations have been shown to have a higher failure rate than was previously quoted[7]. For all these reasons, continued long-term OC use should be discussed as an alternative to tubal sterilization.

OCs also provide prevention and treatment of menstrual cycle disorders such as menstrual irregularity secondary to erratic ovulation, shortened cycles due to a reduced follicular phase, and heavy menses and associated anemia[8–10]. OC use opposes the perimenopausal hyperestrogenic state on the uterine muscle, preventing fibroid growth[11,12]. OCs do not stimulate the growth of fibroids and therefore are not contraindicated in their presence[10–12]. OCs have been shown to decrease the duration of bleeding and increase hematocrit in patients with known leiomyomas[13]. By preventing hormonal fluctuations, patients may experience a decrease in premenstrual symptomatology and sporadic

Table 1 Beneficial effects of perimenopausal use of oral contraceptives

Contraceptive issues
Reduction in unintended pregnancies
Reduction in abortion
Reduction in ectopic pregnancies
Reduced need for sterilization

Benign gynecological disorders
Reduction in irregular menses secondary to erratic
 ovulation
Lengthening of cycles with a shortened follicular phase
Reduction in menstrual blood loss and associated
 anemia
Reduction in ovarian cysts
Reduction in premenstrual symptomatology
Possible reduction in fibroid growth and endometriosis

Estrogen deficiency symptoms/sequelae
Treatment of vasomotor symptoms
Prevention of bone loss
Prevention of rheumatoid arthritis

Effects on the breast
Reduction in fibrocystic masses
Reduction in fibroadenomas

Cancer prevention
Reduction in ovarian cancer
Reduction in endometrial cancer
Possible reduction in colorectal cancer

Diagnostic/therapeutic procedures
Decreased need for endometrial biopsy, curettage,
 hysteroscopy, sonography, ablations and hysterectomy
 for menstrual bleeding disorders
Reduced need for diagnostic laparoscopy and
 hysterectomy for pelvic pain
Reduced need for gynecological oncology procedures
 secondary to malignancies

vasomotor symptoms[8]. By inhibiting ovulation, OCs are also associated with a reduction in functional ovarian cysts and ovarian cancer[14–16]. Ovarian cysts in perimenopausal patients are often cause for concern because of the increased potential of associated malignancies and, although most are functional, they often lead to a quicker decision to pursue surgical diagnosis and treatment. The incidence of endometrial cancer is also reduced in OC users[17,18]. OC use is also associated with a reduction in pelvic pain associated with menses and ovulation[19]. Because of the multitude of effects on the endometrium, myometrium and ovary, gynecological problems are often prevented or adequately treated, reducing the need for diagnostic and therapeutic procedures. Abnormal bleeding often leads to endometrial biopsy, hysteroscopy, sonography, endometrial ablation and even hysterectomy. Pelvic pain often requires diagnostic laparoscopy or hysterectomy. Ovarian and endometrial cancers usually require extensive gynecological surgery. The majority of these benign gynecological conditions and cancers and their associated morbidity and mortality could be avoided with prolonged OC use.

Positive effects of OCs are also seen on the breast, with a reduction in fibrocystic masses and fibroadenomas[20]. Other non-gynecological benefits of OCs have also been suggested. While bone density normally begins to decrease in the late thirties, OC use appears to halt this bone resorption. Several studies have shown an increase in bone mineral density in women using OCs[21–26], and a reduction in hip fractures during the menopause if OCs were used after the age of 40[27]. Other studies have found a reduced rate of arthritis in prior OC users[28,29]. Evidence is also accumulating that OC use may reduce the risk of colorectal cancer[30–33].

Reasons that oral contraceptives are not used in perimenopausal women

Considering the many beneficial effects of OC use, particularly in women in the latter half of their reproductive life, the reasons for lack of use in this age group need to be explored (Table 2). While there are legitimate reasons not to use OCs in some cases, many patients are not offered OCs or decline their use when offered.

Contraindications of OC use in women of all ages include a personal history of thromboembolic events, myocardial infarction, cerebrovascular accidents, breast cancer and severe liver disease. In women over the age of 35, other factors should be considered. Patients with risk factors for cardiovascular

Table 2 Reasons that oral contraceptives are not used in perimenopausal women

Contraindications
Side-effects
Provider fear/concerns
Patient fear/concerns
Compliance
Costs

disease are not ideal OC candidates. These risk factors include smoking, hypertension, morbid obesity, diabetes and cholesterol abnormalities. When these risks are multiple and/or not well controlled, manifestations of cardiovascular disease are more likely to present themselves in women in their forties and early fifties. An increased risk of myocardial infarction is seen in patients on OCs with a history of high blood pressure[34]. The combination of smoking and OC use has also been associated with increased cardiovascular disease, especially with increased reproductive age[35–38]. Hence, most practitioners consider OC use a contraindication in women over the age of 35 who smoke. A good rule of thumb is that OC use in women in their forties and fifties should be limited to healthy non-smokers.

Side-effects are a common reason that OCs are not used in the perimenopause. When recommended as a treatment option, patients often reply 'I can't take the pill' and list numerous side-effects such as nausea, headaches and mood swings when they had attempted the pill many years previously. Fortunately, there are now pills and other methods of taking it that have fewer side-effects. In a study published by Sulak and colleagues in 2000[39], side-effects such as headaches, pain, breast tenderness and bloating/swelling were observed more often during the 7-day hormone-free interval than during the 21-day active-pill period. The 7-day hormone-free interval not only creates hormone withdrawal symptoms during that week but also creates problems in the next cycle. At the end of the hormone-free week, FSH levels begin to rise and ovarian hormone production increases into the next cycle. Spona and co-workers[40] showed that decreasing the hormone-free interval from 7 to 5 days provided greater ovarian inhibition. There is now one OC on the market in the USA that has only 2 hormone-free days followed by 5 days of ethinyl estradiol 10 μg[41] (Mircette®; Organon Inc., West Orange, NJ). Using lower-dose pills may also decrease side-effects. In a randomized study of two 20-μg OCs and one triphasic 30-μg OC, the 20-μg OCs had fewer side-effects[42]. Counselling is critical in this age group, particularly in relation to side-effects. Patients should understand that almost all women will experience at least one side-effect upon initiation of OCs; these include nausea, headaches, mood swings, breakthrough bleeding/breakthrough spotting, breast tenderness and bloating/swelling. However, these side-effects spontaneously resolve in most patients during the first one to three cycles. Patients need to be counselled that, if side-effects persist, they should record exactly when the side-effects occur during the pill cycle. If the side-effects occur during the last week of the active-pill period and into the hormone-free interval, the 21-day/7-day regimen can be altered to decrease or eliminate their occurrence.

OCs are often not recommended to women over the age of 40, even if it is the treatment of choice, because of provider fears and concerns. In most OC studies, patients over the age of 40 are excluded. Several articles have been published on women over the age of 40 taking OCs, and when subjects were limited to healthy non-smokers, complications did not occur[8,21,43]. OCs do increase the risk of venous thrombosis from a baseline risk of less than 1 per 10 000 person-years in non-users to 3–4 per 10 000 person-years in OC users[44,45]. Rarely are these venous thrombosis events fatal. In a World Health Organization report on hormonal contraception and myocardial infarction, non-smoking, normotensive, non-diabetic women of any age who used OCs were found not to be at increased risk of myocardial infarction compared with non-users[45]. In a recent study, risk of myocardial

Table 3 Myths surrounding oral contraceptives

The pill causes cancer
One can be on the pill too long
The pill is dangerous
One can be too old to be on the pill
The pill causes weight gain

infarction was increased among women using second-generation OCs (levonorgestrel) but not third-generation OCs (desogestrel)[46]. Ischemic or hemorrhagic stroke does not appear to be increased in healthy non-smoking OC users[45,47]. Smoking, hypertension and a history of migraines are associated with an increase in the relative risk of stroke among OC users[36,45,47,48]. When considering the risks versus benefits of OC use, the benefits far outweigh the risks in healthy normotensive non-smokers.

Patients also have fears that are not substantiated but must be addressed (Table 3). These myths regarding OC use can affect patient initiation and compliance. Patients fear that the pill will cause cancer and need to be informed that it actually reduces the risk of endometrial and ovarian cancer. Data on OC use and breast cancer are reassuring[49,50]. In a large collaborative reanalysis, ever-users of OCs had a relative risk of breast cancer of 1.06 compared with never-users[49]. This was an observational study, and such a small increase in risk is difficult to interpret. The authors suggested that the small increase in risk may have been due to increased monitoring, with earlier diagnosis of breast cancer in OC users. The data suggested that much of the increased risk of breast cancer found in recent OC users was due to an increased diagnosis of localized tumors, rather than diagnosis of invasive disease spread beyond the breast. In this study, OC users had a statistically significant decrease in metastatic breast disease. The reanalysis demonstrated that estrogen dose, progestin type or dose and duration of use did not affect the risk of breast cancer. Also, OC use did not increase breast cancer risk in women with a family history of breast cancer[49].

Patients must also be reassured of the safety of OC use if they remain healthy non-smokers. Risks of use in this setting are rare, especially compared with the benefits. The safety of long-term use must also be addressed. While no studies have been published implicating long-term use and greater complications, many studies have documented the benefits of long-term use to include reduction in cancer, prevention of menstrual disorders and maintenance of bone mineral density. While some medications today are associated with serious complications, especially if used for years, complications of OCs such as thromboembolic events generally occur in the first year of use. The benefits and safety of long-term OC use, even for decades, are not commonly appreciated by patients and need to be emphasized. Patients are also concerned that the pill may cause significant weight gain. A pooled analysis from two placebo-controlled OC trials found the same weight gain in the placebo and OC users[51]. A new 30 μg ethinyl estradiol OC containing drosperinone has been associated with weight *loss* in the first 6–9 months of use[52,53].

Daily compliance is often listed as a reason for not wanting to initiate OCs. Patients may relate that they do not want to take a pill every day or have trouble taking a pill every day. This is where education is vital. If patients are fully aware of the benefits to be gained from OC use, adherence to a regimen will be inherently reinforced. This age group also needs to be informed of the needs for daily calcium supplementation and the concept that, as one ages, medications are often recommended as a preventive therapy. OCs fall into this category and can be described as the best 'supplement' available today.

Unfortunately, cost is still an issue for many patients and can affect initiation and continuation. The multitude of benefits of prolonged OC use make it a highly cost-effective medication by decreasing pain and bleeding, which often require other associated expenses.

Counselling about oral contraceptives

When initiating OCs in perimenopausal women, appropriate counselling is critical and age-specific (Table 4). A detailed medical history is important, to ensure that the patient is a healthy non-smoker with no history of thromboembolic events. If there are no contraindications, it is important to spend a few minutes discussing all of the benefits of OCs and how the pill can impact her health not only immediately but years after discontinuation. By educating the perimenopausal woman on the health issues of declining, fluctuating ovarian function and how the pill has the potential to resolve these problems along with supplying many other benefits, initiation of OCs is more likely to occur, even in patients who initially may be extremely opposed to the concept. Dispelling the many OC myths previously discussed will also allay unsubstantiated fears and encourage the patient to attempt a trial of OCs.

The patient must also understand that nuisance side-effects are common and occur to some extent in almost all patients during the initial cycles. A discussion of all possible side-effects is critical to prevent unnecessary alarm when they occur. If patients are fully aware of the benefits and that side-effects are common and usually spontaneously resolve or can be managed they are more apt to continue OCs. Having the patient commit to a 3-month trial of therapy is important prior to initiation. A discussion of all possible serious complications associated with the pill, particularly thromboembolic events, is important.

If the patient wishes to initiate OCs after ruling out contraindications and discussing non-contraceptive benefits, myths, side-effects and possible complications, a review of OC packaging is important, as most perimenopausal patients have not taken OCs for many years. Patients may need assistance in determining what time of day to take their pill and where to place them in order to maintain strict daily compliance. Starting OCs within the first

Table 4 Recommended counselling about oral contraceptives (OCs)

Rule out contraindications
Emphasize non-contraceptive benefits
Dispel the myths
Detail the nuisance side-effects
Review rare complications
Review OC packaging
Encourage strict compliance
Discuss alternative regimens

day or two of menses may provide greater follicular control in that cycle, as opposed to starting later in the cycle, thus reducing the risk of bothersome breakthrough bleeding and spotting. A follow-up appointment towards the end of the second pack or during the third cycle is often the key to continued adherence to OC use. During the visit, blood pressure can be reassessed and side-effects discussed. It is important that the patient is asked whether side-effects such as bloating/swelling, breast tenderness and headaches occur at the end of the active-pill period and into the hormone-free interval. The regimen can be altered to eliminate or reduce these estrogen withdrawal symptoms. In a study of hormone withdrawal symptoms during the OC hormone-free interval, patients were offered extension of their active tablets to up to 12 consecutive weeks[54]. Seventy-four per cent opted for the extended regimen. In a follow-up study, 292 patients were given the option of altering their 21-day/7-day regimen of OCs by extending the active-pill period and reducing the 7-day hormone-free interval[55]. Ninety-two per cent attempted extension, with approximately 60% continuing to extend at the time of follow-up. The average number of weeks of consecutive active pills was 12, with a maximum of 102 consecutive weeks. The average hormone-free interval was 5 days, with a range of 0–7 days. In this study of 292 patients, 101 were aged 40 or more years. Since hormone withdrawal symptoms are so common, varied and often severe in OC users, discussing their occurrence is important so that the patient can recognize and report the nature and timing of side-effects. Extending the active-pill period and reducing the hormone-free interval should be considered in all perimenopausal patients on OCs. A study of menstrual frequency preferences revealed that the majority of older reproductive-aged women preferred menses every 3 months to never[56]. Altering the 21-day/7-day regimen allows patients the convenience of infrequent menses and avoidance of numerous side-effects. Two approaches can be used in counselling patients on extending their active-pill period. Patients can be instructed to take the pill consecutively for a desired number of weeks, such as 6, 9 or 12, followed by a 4–7-day hormone-free interval. Alternatively, patients can be instructed to continue taking pills until some bleeding occurs, to then stop taking the pills for 3–4 days, and then to resume. For many patients this is an ideal method, because many perimenopausal patients have severe estrogen withdrawal symptoms such as mood swings and headaches if they have a 7-day hormone-free interval. This allows them to take the pills often for months at a time, followed by a reduced hormone-free interval to prevent the occurrence of estrogen withdrawal symptoms. To date, no data have been published on extending the number of pills of a 20-μg OC. Theoretically, more breakthrough bleeding may occur when attempting to extend a 20-μg OC compared with a 30-μg OC[57]. Since there are no advantages to triphasic pills over monophasic pills, and extension of the active-pill period should be an option given to perimenopausal women, use of monophasic pills is recommended. If a patient is on a triphasic pill and continuous use of OCs is being considered, the patient can easily be converted to the 20–30-μg equivalent pill and counselled on the benefits of changing her current OC and altering the current 21-day/7-day regimen. If she is on a 20-μg OC and breakthrough spotting/bleeding occurs, she can be converted to a monophasic 30-μg OC. Future studies with alterations in the 21-day/7-day design will elucidate preferred methods of extending the active-pill period. An OC with 84 active pills is currently being researched (Barr Laboratories, New York).

Switching from oral contraceptives to hormone replacement therapy

When to switch a patient from OCs to hormone replacement therapy is often a dilemma for many practitioners. Since the median age of menopause is almost 52 years, if OCs are stopped prior to that age, half the women will still not be menopausal[58]. Stopping OCs prematurely may put the patient at risk for the numerous problems outlined during the perimenopausal phase of fluctuating ovarian function. If the patient remains a healthy non-smoker and is doing well on OCs, taking them in the standard or extended-cycle fashion, then continuing OCs until approximately the age of 55 will ensure that the majority of women have gone through the menopause and hormone replacement therapy can be started at that time. If the patient resumes monthly menses spontaneously after discontinuing OCs, the OCs can be reinitiated for another year. Alternatively, FSH levels can be assessed at the end of the hormone-free interval to diagnose menopause[59–61]. An FSH level of > 20 mIU/ml suggests, but does not guarantee, complete cessation of ovulation and menses.

Summary

The perimenopause is fraught with a multitude of gynecological disorders (physical and emotional) secondary to declining erratic ovarian function. OCs are the mainstay of therapy for these problems in healthy non-smokers. They are greatly underutilized in this age group for the reasons outlined. Greater use of OCs will prevent or treat many of the disorders discussed, thereby decreasing the morbidity and mortality associated with these problems. Altering the 21-day/7-day OC regimen has the potential to reduce side-effects and improve compliance, allowing perimenopausal women to benefit from the numerous advantages of OC use.

References

1. Santoro N, Brown JR, Adel T, *et al*. Characterization of reproductive hormonal dynamics in the perimenopause. *J Clin Endocrinol Metab* 1996;81:1495–501

2. Henshaw SK. Unintended pregnancy in the United States. *Fam Plann Perspect* 1998;30:24–9

3. Stergachis A, Shy KK, Grothaus LC, *et al*. Tubal sterilization and the long-term risk of hysterectomy. *J Am Med Assoc* 1990;264:2893–8

4. Rubin MC, Davidson AR, Philliber SG, *et al*. Long-term effect of tubal sterilization on menstrual indices and pelvic pain. *Obstet Gynecol* 1993;82:118–21

5. Hillis SD, Marchbanks PA, Tylor LR, *et al*., for the U.S. Collaborative Review of Sterilization Working Group. Higher hysterectomy risk for sterilized than nonsterilized women: findings from the U.S. Collaborative Review of Sterilization. *Obstet Gynecol* 1998;91:241–6

6. Schmidt JE, Hillis SD, Marchbanks PA, *et al*., for the U.S. Collaborative Review of Sterilization Working Group. Requesting information about and obtaining reversal after tubal sterilization: findings from the U.S. collaborative review. *Fertil Steril* 2000;74:892–8

7. Petersen HB, Xia Z, Hughes JM, *et al*., for the U.S. Collaborative Review of Sterilization Working Group. The risk of pregnancy after tubal sterilization. *Am J Obstet Gynecol* 1996;174:1161–70

8. Casper RF, Dodin S, Reid RL, *et al*. The effect of 20-mcg ethinyl estradiol/1 mg norethindrone acetate (Minestrin™), a low-dose oral contraceptive, on vaginal bleeding patterns, hot flashes, and quality of life in symptomatic perimenopausal women. *Menopause* 1997;4:139–47

9. Davis A, Godwin A, Lippman J, *et al*. Triphasic norgestimate–ethinyl estradiol for treating dysfunctional uterine bleeding. *Obstet Gynecol* 2000;96:913–20

10. Friedman AJ, Thomas PP. Does low-dose combination oral contraceptive use affect uterine size or menstrual flow in premenopausal women with leiomyomas? *Obstet Gynecol* 1995;85:631–5

11. Ross RK, Pike MC, Vessey MP, *et al*. Risk factors for uterine fibroids: reduced risk associated with oral contraceptives. *Br Med J* 1986;293:359–62

12. Parazzini F, Negri E, LaVecchia C, *et al*. Oral contraceptive use and the risk of fibroids. *Obstet Gynecol* 1992;79:430–3

13. Larsson G, Milsom I, Lindstedt G, *et al*. The influence of a low-dose combined oral contraceptive on menstrual blood loss and iron status. *Contraception* 1992;46:327–34

14. Hankinson SE, Colditz GA, Hunter DJ, *et al*. A quantitative assessment of oral contraceptive use and risk of ovarian cancer. *Obstet Gynecol* 1992;80:708–14

15. The Cancer and Steroid Hormone Study of the Centers for Disease Control and the National Institute of Child Health and Human Development. The reduction in risk of ovarian cancer associated with oral-contraceptive use. *N Engl J Med* 1987;316:650–5

16. Ness RB, Grisso JA, Klapper J, *et al*. Risk of ovarian cancer in relation to estrogen and progestin dose and use characteristics of oral contraceptives. *Am J Epidemiol* 2000;152:233–41

17. Schlesselman JJ. Risk of endometrial cancer in relation to use of combined oral contraceptives; a practitioner's guide to meta-analysis. *Hum Reprod* 1997;12:1851–63

18. The Cancer and Steroid Hormone Study of the Centers for Disease Control and the National Institute of Child Health and Human Development. Combination oral contraceptive use and the risk of endometrial cancer. *J Am Med Assoc* 1987;257:796–800

19. Milsom I, Sundell G, Andersch B. The influence of different combined oral contraceptives on the prevalence and severity of dysmenorrhea. *Contraception* 1990;42:497–506

20. Charreau I, Plu-Bureau G, Bachelot A, *et al*. Oral contraceptive use and the risk of benign breast disease in a French case–control study. *Eur J Cancer Prev* 1993;2:147–54

21. Gambacciani M, Spinetti A, Cappagli B, *et al*. Hormone replacement therapy in perimenopausal women with a low dose oral contraceptive preparation: effects on bone mineral density and metabolism. *Maturitas* 1994;19:125–31

22. Kleerekoper M, Brienza RS, Schultz LR, *et al*. Oral contraceptive use may protect against low bone mass. *Arch Intern Med* 1991;151:1971–6

23. Kritz-Silverstein D, Barrett-Connor E. Bone mineral density in postmenopausal women as determined by prior oral contraceptive use. *Am J Public Health* 1993;83:100–2

24. Pasco JA, Kotowicz MA, Henry MJ, *et al*. Oral contraceptives and bone mineral density: a population-based study. *Am J Obstet Gynecol* 2000;182:265–9

25. Petitti DB, Piaggio G, Mehta S, *et al*. Steroid hormone contraception and bone mineral density:

a cross-sectional study in an international population. *Obstet Gynecol* 2000;95:736–44

26. DeCherney A. Bone-sparing properties of oral contraceptives. *Am J Obstet Gynecol* 1996;174: 15–20

27. Michäelsson K, Baron JS, Farahmand BY, *et al.* Oral-contraceptive use and risk of hip fracture: a case–control study. *Lancet* 1999;353: 1481–4

28. Spector TD, Hochberg MC. The protective effect of the oral contraceptive pill on rheumatoid arthritis: an overview of the analytic epidemiological studies using meta-analysis. *J Clin Epidemiol* 1990;43:1221–30

29. Jorgensen C, Picot MC, Bologna C, *et al.* Oral contraception, parity, breast feeding, and severity of rheumatoid arthritis. *Ann Rheum Dis* 1996;55:94–8

30. Fernandez E, La Vecchia C, Francheschi S, *et al.* Oral contraceptive use and risk of colorectal cancer. *Epidemiology* 1998;9:295–300

31. Potter JD, McMichael AJ. Large bowel cancer in women in relation to reproductive and hormonal factors: a case–control study. *J Natl Cancer Inst* 1983;71:703–9

32. Martinez MD, Grodstein F, Giovannucci E, *et al.* A prospective study of reproductive factors, oral contraceptive use, and risk of colorectal cancer. *Cancer Epidemiol Biomarkers Prev* 1997; 6:1–5

33. Fernandez E, LaVecchia C, Balducci A, *et al.* Oral contraceptives and colorectal cancer risk: a meta-analysis. *Br J Cancer* 2001;84:722–7

34. Croft P, Hannaford PC. Risk factors for acute myocardial infarction in women: evidence from the Royal College of General Practitioners' Oral Contraceptive Study. *Br Med J* 1989;298:165–8

35. Rosenberg L, Palmer JR, Lesko SM, Shapiro S. Oral contraceptive use and the risk of myocardial infraction. *Am J Epidemiol* 1990;131: 1009–16

36. WHO Collaborative Study of Cardiovascular Disease and Steroid Hormone Contraception. Ischaemic stroke and combined oral contraceptives: results of an international, multicentre case–control study. *Lancet* 1996;348: 498–505

37. WHO Collaborative Study of Cardiovascular Disease and Steroid Hormone Contraception. Acute myocardial infarction and combined oral contraceptives: results of an international multicentre case–control study. *Lancet* 1997;349:1202–9

38. Fruzzetti F, Ricci C, Fioretti P. Haemostasis profile in smoking and nonsmoking women taking low-dose oral contraceptives. *Contraception* 1994;49:579–92

39. Sulak PJ, Scow RD, Preece C, *et al.* Hormone withdrawal symptoms in oral contraceptive users. *Obstet Gynecol* 2000;95:261–6

40. Spona J, Elstein M, Feichtinger W, *et al.* Shorter pill-free interval in combined oral contraceptives decreases follicular development. *Contraception* 1996;53:71–7

41. Killick SR, Fitzgerald C, Davis A. Ovarian activity in women taking an oral contraceptive containing 20 μg ethinyl estradiol and 150 μg desogestrel: effects of low dose estrogen during the hormone-free interval. *Am J Obstet Gynecol* 1998;179:518–24

42. Rosenberg MJ, Myers A, Roy V. Efficacy, cycle control, and side effects of low- and lower-dose oral contraceptives: a randomized trial of 20 mg and 35 mg estrogen preparations. *Contraception* 1999;60:321–9

43. Shargil AA. Hormone replacement therapy in perimenopausal women with a triphasic contraceptive compound: a three-year prospective study. *Int J Fertil* 1985;30:15–28

44. Vandenbroucke JP, Rosing J, Bloemenkamp KW, *et al.* Oral contraceptives and the risk of venous thrombosis. *N Engl J Med* 2001;344: 1527–34

45. World Health Organization. Report of a WHO Scientific Group. *Cardiovascular Disease and Steroid Hormone Contraception*. WHO Technical Bulletin Series 877. Geneva: WHO, 1998

46. Tanis BC, van den Bosch MA, Kemmeren JM, *et al.* Oral contraceptives and the risk of myocardial infarction. *N Engl J Med* 2001;345: 1787–93

47. Schwartz SM, Petitti DB, Siscovick DS, *et al.* Stroke and use of low-dose oral contraceptives in young women: a pooled analysis of two US studies. *Stroke* 1998;29:2277–84

48. Chang CL, Donaghy M, Poulter N, *et al.* Migraine and stroke in young women: case–control study. *Br Med J* 1999;318:13–18

49. Collaborative Group on Hormonal Factors in Breast Cancer. Breast cancer and hormonal contraceptives: further results. *Contraception* 1996;54(Suppl):1S–106S

50. Rosenberg L, Palmer JR, Rao RS, *et al.* Case–control study of oral contraceptive use and risk of breast cancer. *Am J Epidemiol* 1996;143:25–37

51. Redmond G, Godwin AJ, Olson W, *et al.* Use of placebo controls in an oral contraceptive trial: methodological issues and adverse event incidence. *Contraception* 1999;60:81–5

52. Parsey K, Pong A. An open-label, multicenter study to evaluate Yasmin, a low-dose combination oral contraceptive containing drospirenone, a new progestogen. *Contraception* 2000;61: 105–11

53. Foidart JM, Wurrke W, Bouw GM, *et al.* A comparative investigation of contraceptive reliability, cycle control and tolerance of two monophasic oral contraceptives containing either drospirenone or desogestrel. *Eur J Contracept Reprod Healthcare* 2000;5:124–34

54. Sulak PJ, Creasman BE, Waldrop E, *et al.* Extending the duration of active oral contraceptive pills to manage hormone withdrawal symptoms. *Obstet Gynecol* 1997;89:179–83

55. Sulak PJ, Kuehl TJ, Ortiz M, *et al.* Acceptance of altering the standard 21 day/7 day oral contraceptive regimen to delay menses and reduce hormone withdrawal symptoms. *Am J Obstet Gynecol* 2002;186:1142–9

56. den Tonkelaar I, Oddens BJ. Preferred frequency and characteristics of menstrual bleeding in relation to reproductive status, oral contraceptive use, and hormone replacement therapy use. *Contraception* 1999;59:357–62

57. Sulak P, Lippman J, Siu C, *et al.* Clinical comparison of triphasic norgestimate/35 μg ethinyl estradiol and monophasic norethindrone acetate/20 μg ethinyl estradiol: cycle conrol, lipid effects, and user satisfaction. *Contraception* 1999;59:161–6

58. McKinlay SM, Brambilla DJ, Posner JG. The normal menopause transition. *Maturitas* 1992; 14:103–15

59. Speroff L. Menopause and the perimenopausal transition. In Speroff L, Glass RH, Kase NG, eds. *Clinical Gynecologic Endocrinology and Infertility*, 6th edn. Philadelphia, PA: Lippincott Williams and Wilkins,1999:643–724

60. Castracane VD, Gimpel T, Goldzieher JW. When is it safe to switch from oral contraceptives to hormonal replacement therapy? *Contraception* 1995;52:371–6

61. Creinin MD. Laboratory criteria for menopause in women using oral contraceptives. *Fertil Steril* 1996;66:101–4

Reduction of breast cancer risk in midlife women

12

S. R. Goldstein

Approximately 180 000 new cases of breast cancer are diagnosed annually in the USA[1]. In addition, there are approximately 45 000 deaths. The case fatality rate for breast cancer is relatively high compared with other cancers, except for those of the lung and ovary. However, the perceptions of women concerning breast cancer are out of proportion to the reality. In 1995, a Gallup poll, commissioned by the North American Menopause Society, queried women about the diseases they believed to be the most common causes of death among women. Forty per cent of those surveyed believed it to be breast cancer. In reality, the lifetime risk of death due to breast cancer is 3.6% or 1/28[2]. Nonetheless, it remains the second most common malignancy in women after lung cancer. The emotional and psychological ramifications of developing breast cancer, and the concomitant fear of the disease, are overwhelming for many women.

Perimenopausal women are particularly susceptible to these fears. Most have already had their families and/or plateaued in their career aspirations. Stress from children entering adolescence and/or their own parents requiring increasing attention and assistance contribute to an overall increase in a woman's concern for her own health. Illness and death among peers, as well as overall life experience, lead to women in this age group beginning to confront their own mortality. Furthermore, there are objective and quantifiable reasons for perimenopausal women's increasing fear about development of breast cancer. Between 1970 and 1990, the number of cases of invasive breast cancer in women under the age of 40 reported to the SEER Program doubled[3]. However, in that same time period (1970–90) the overall number of women in the USA aged 35–39 increased by only about 50%.

In the past, major efforts were directed at early detection of breast cancer mainly because of the belief that this would have a positive impact on the outcome, and thus also improve survival. Established factors that influence breast cancer risk[4] include: increasing age, early menarche, late menopause, proliferative breast disease, family history of breast cancer, *BRCA1* or *BRCA2* mutations, late first-term pregnancy or nulliparity, North American or Western European background, mammographic pattern of increased density and ionizing radiation exposure. Relative risks for various breast cancer risk factors are shown in Table 1.

A woman's decisions relative to her breast health – whether she undergoes a program of intensive surveillance with mammography and ultrasound, considers chemopreventive agents, or possibly even undergoes prophylactic mastectomy – critically depends on her awareness of the medical options, her own personal preferences and, importantly, an individualized estimate of the probability of her developing breast cancer over a defined period of time. Such an estimate is also useful for designing prevention trials in high-risk subsets of the population. Prevention trials differ from therapeutic clinical trials in that asymptomatic healthy women are exposed to potentially toxic interventions for prolonged periods of time, in order to reduce the risk of developing breast cancer. Risk estimates for various individual risk factors are available (Table 1) but risk estimates for combinations of risk factors are clearly preferable. The Gail

Table 1 Breast cancer risk factors and their relative risks. Adapted from reference 5

Relative risk < 2
Age 25–34 at first live birth
Early menarche
Late menopause
Proliferative benign disease
Postmenopausal obesity
Alcohol use
Hormone replacement therapy

Relative risk 2–4
Age > 35 at first live birth
First-degree relative with breast cancer
Nulliparity
Radiation exposure
Prior breast cancer

Relative risk > 4
Gene mutations
Lobular carcinoma *in situ*
Ductal carcinoma *in situ*
Atypical hyplasia

---

model[6] takes into account some non-genetic factors (e.g. nulliparity, age at menarche, pre-existing pathological conditions) as well as genetic factors (family history). The model calculates a woman's individualized breast cancer probability and yields a percentage risk of developing invasive breast cancer over the following 5 years as well as for the remainder of her expected lifetime.

There are limitations to the Gail model's approach to estimating the risk of breast cancer. The Gail model uses the number of previous breast biopsies in its calculation of risk assessment. The relative risk associated with the previous breast biopsy is lower for women over the age of 50 than it is for younger women. Furthermore, the data from which Gail made these assessments were collected in the late 1970s and early 1980s. Increasing ease of breast histopathological assessment through fine-needle aspiration and outpatient core-needle biopsy creates tremendous confusion for the clinician in understanding what exactly constitutes a 'breast biopsy'.

Therefore, the 1.66% risk over the next 5 years, adopted as a cut-off to determine 'high risk' for the Breast Cancer Prevention Trial

(BCPT) run by the National Surgical Adjuvant Breast and Bowel Project (NSABP; see below), becomes somewhat more difficult to interpret in the light of current practice. Consider the following example. A 50-year-old nulliparous Caucasian woman with menarche at age 11, with no first-degree relatives in her family who have had breast cancer, and who has never had any breast biopsies, has a Gail model calculated risk of developing breast cancer of 1.2% in the next 5 years and 10.8% in her lifetime. She is not labelled as 'high risk'. If the same patient were to give a history of three previous breast biopsies, none of which were hyperplastic, her risk would be calculated at 1.8% over 5 years and 15.8% in her lifetime. This falls into the high-risk category. To most patients any histological sampling of the breast constitutes a biopsy. With increasing ease of obtaining such material the utilization of the biopsy has increased. Practice patterns can, therefore, alter risk estimates substantially.

Identification of objective findings that are patient-specific but highly correlative with development of breast cancer would be clearly desirable. Patient-specific biomarkers have been proposed[7]. An example would be ultrasensitive measurement of serum estradiol levels in postmenopausal women to identify those at higher risk of developing breast cancer. In the Multiple Outcomes of Raloxifene Evaluation (MORE) trial, those women who experienced the greatest reduction in breast cancer during treatment with raloxifene were those with the highest baseline levels of serum estradiol (Figure 1), although overall all patients were well within the postmenopausal range (≤ 20 pmol/l)[7].

Rationale for tamoxifen in breast cancer prevention

The theory behind using tamoxifen for primary prevention of breast cancer in healthy women has its roots in preclinical animal and *in vitro* studies. Tamoxifen inhibited mammary tumors in mice and rats, and suppressed

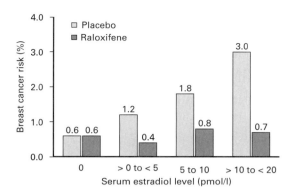

Figure 1 Risk of breast cancer over 4 years, shown among patients in the placebo and raloxifene groups with various baseline serum concentrations of estradiol. From reference 8

Table 2 Tamoxifen and contralateral breast cancer: overview analysis. Adapted from reference 11

	Reduction (%)	p Value
Duration (years)		
1	13	NS
2	26	0.004
5	47	0.00001
Age (years)		
≤ 50	27	
> 50	31	
ER status		
ER positive	30	
ER poor	29	

ER, estrogen receptor

hormone-dependent breast cancer cell lines *in vitro*[9]. The clinical data from the Early Breast Cancer Trialists' Collaborative Group[10] gave additional motivation for prevention trials with tamoxifen. In addition to the reduction in recurrent breast cancer, tamoxifen reduced the risk of contralateral new-onset breast cancer by 47% after 5 years of adjuvant treatment (Table 2). Thus, the preclinical *in vitro* and animal models coupled with clinical data, together with tamoxifen's favorable effects on skeleton remodelling and lipid levels, led to the development of a series of chemopreventive trials using tamoxifen in both the USA and Europe (Table 3).

Breast Cancer Prevention Trial

The NSABP launched a prevention trial using tamoxifen in 1992. A total of 13 388 women aged 35 or older, who were deemed to be at high risk for breast cancer, were enrolled at numerous sites throughout the USA and Canada. The Gail model[6] was used to determine women whose breast cancer risk was judged sufficient to warrant inclusion in the trial. Women needed to have a risk of developing invasive breast cancer within the following 5 years of 1.66% or greater to be included. Patients were randomly assigned to receive placebo or tamoxifen 20 mg/day for 5 years. The trial was terminated early, in April 1998, because of the dramatic reduction in new-onset breast cancer with tamoxifen relative to placebo (Figure 2).

The overall incidence of breast cancer in the tamoxifen group was 3.4 cases/1000 compared with a breast cancer incidence in the placebo group of 6.8 cases/1000[12]. Overall the reduction in invasive breast cancer was 49% ($p < 0.00001$). When broken down into various age groups, the reduction was 44% in women aged 35–49 years, 51% in women aged 50–59 years and 55% in women aged 60 years and older (Figure 3).

In the BCPT, tamoxifen decreased the incidence of non-invasive breast cancer (ductal carcinoma *in situ*) by 50%. The expanded use of mammography has resulted in the increased frequency of detection of ductal carcinoma *in situ*. Most ductal carcinoma *in situ* lesions have been demonstrated to be estrogen receptor-positive[13]. In addition, in the BCPT, tamoxifen reduced breast cancer risk in women with a history of lobular carcinoma *in situ* by 56% and atypical hyperplasia by 86%. Overall, tamoxifen decreased the occurrence of estrogen receptor-positive tumors by 69%, but had no impact on the incidence of estrogen receptor-negative tumors.

The BCPT was stopped 14 months before its planned completion because the data and safety monitoring board felt that it was unethical to continue to allow one-half of the participants, deemed to be at high risk for

Table 3 Tamoxifen prevention trials

	NSABP[10]	Royal Marsden[12]	Italian[13]
Number of participants	13 388	2471	5408
Age ≤ 50 years	40%	62%	36%
One first-degree relative with breast cancer	55%	55%	18%
Two or more first-degree relatives with breast cancer	13%	17%	2.5%
Hormone replacement therapy users	0%	42%	8%
Woman-years of follow-up	46 858	12 355	20 731
Cancer incidence/1000			
placebo	6.8	5.0	2.3
tamoxifen	3.4	4.7	2.1

NSABP, National Surgical Adjuvant Breast and Bowel Project

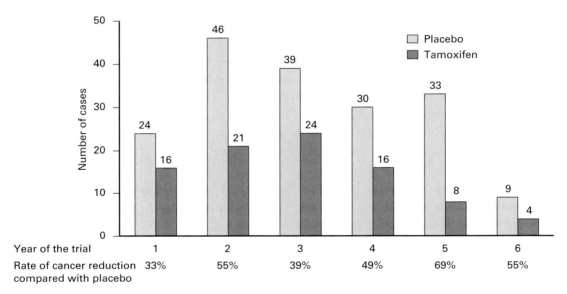

Figure 2 Number of cases of breast cancer in the Breast Cancer Prevention Trial. Adapted from reference 12

developing breast cancer, to continue to take placebo in light of the dramatic reduction by tamoxifen in both invasive and non invasive breast cancer.

Royal Marsden Trial

This was one of two European tamoxifen breast cancer prevention trials that did not confirm the BCPT results[14]. This British trial studied 2471 healthy women between the ages of 30 and 70 years who had a family history of breast cancer. The immediate follow-up was 70 months. There was no statistically significant decrease in breast cancer with tamoxifen use compared with placebo. One possibility for the discrepancy with the BCPT may be that eligibility for the Royal Marsden Trial was based predominantly on a strong family history of breast cancer. Furthermore, a much larger number of women were younger than 50 years of age (62%, compared with only about 40% of the BCPT). Finally, 42% of the women received

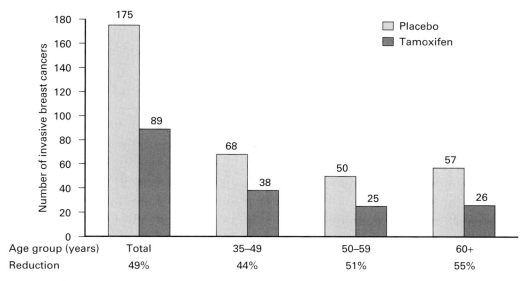

Figure 3 Number of invasive breast cancers in the Breast Cancer Prevention Trial

concomitant hormone replacement therapy along with tamoxifen during that trial.

Italian Tamoxifen Prevention Study

The Italian Tamoxifen Prevention Study also did not confirm the results of the BCPT[15]. This study recruited participants from the general population and therefore their overall risk of breast cancer was significantly lower. Compliance rates in the Italian study were quite low, with approximately 26% of the subjects discontinuing the trial. Finally, the Italian trial had considerably fewer women more than 60 years of age (12% compared with the BCPT 30%).

Effect of tamoxifen on healthy women

The BCPT made available, for the first time, large-scale information about the effects of tamoxifen on healthy women. Previously, all studies of tamoxifen had been in women with breast cancer. Several secondary endpoints are worthy of consideration. The overall relative risk (RR) of endometrial cancer associated with tamoxifen therapy in healthy women was 2.53 (95% confidence interval (CI) 1.35–4.97). However when further analyzed by age, the RR in women > 50 years old was 4.01 (95% CI 1.70–10.90), whereas the RR in women aged ≤ 49 years was 1.21 (95% CI 0.41–3.60). The same age distinction was true for thromboembolic events in terms of deep vein thrombosis and pulmonary emboli. There were no statistically significant increases in pulmonary emboli or deep vein thrombosis in women ≤ 49 years of age. It is unclear whether the trial was sufficiently powered for this particular secondary endpoint. Still, on the basis of these findings, the concerns that serious adverse events with tamoxifen chemoprevention may diminish the potential benefit do not seem to be as powerful in those women < 50 years of age as they are for those women > 50 years of age. This has significant clinical consequences for physicians caring for perimenopausal patients.

Overall, invasive cancers other than those of the breast and uterus were exactly the same in the tamoxifen and the placebo groups. The RR of death from any cause was 0.81 (95% CI 0.56–1.16). There was a slight increase in the risk of myocardial infarction (RR 1.11; 95% CI 0.65–1.92) and a slight decrease in the development of severe angina (RR 0.93; 95% CI 0.40–2.14) in tamoxifen users, although neither of these was statistically significant. In terms of fractures at various sites (hip, spine, radius) the overall RR was 0.81 (95% CI 0.63–1.05). There was a statistically significant increase in the number of women with cataracts who then underwent cataract surgery. That RR was 1.57 (95% CI 1.16–2.14).

Clinical use

In October 1998, based on the BCPT results, the US Food and Drug Administration (FDA) approved tamoxifen for the primary prevention of breast cancer in women at high risk for the disease. It recommended that the use of tamoxifen be limited to high-risk women because of the potentially serious side-effects seen in the clinical trials and discussed above. The FDA did not actually determine high risk but it did make the recommendation that the decision to use tamoxifen as a prophylactic chemopreventive therapy needed to depend on a thorough evaluation of a woman's personal, family and medical histories, her age and her understanding of the assessment of the risks and benefits of treatment.

Although the FDA did not specifically define 'high risk', it required the inclusion of the following passage in the package insert: 'You should not take tamoxifen to reduce the risk of breast cancer unless you are at high risk of breast cancer. Certain conditions put women at high risk and it is possible to calculate this risk for any woman. Breast cancer risk assessment tools to help calculate your risk of breast cancer have been developed and are available to your health care professional. You should discuss your risk with your health care professional.'

BRCA1 and *BRCA2*

There are several forms of familial breast cancer[16]. Familial early-onset breast–ovarian cancer is an autosomal dominant disease that usually affects those at risk before 50 years of age and is typically due to *BRCA1* mutation. Breast cancer without ovarian cancer can be seen in families as well, and is associated with either *BRCA1* or *BRCA2* mutations. This form of disease also has an early onset and is associated with male breast cancer in families with *BRCA2* mutations.

These genes were discovered by collecting DNA from large extended families with an apparent autosomal dominant pattern of inheritance of breast cancer. This led to the identification of polymorphic markers on chromosome 17q21 and on chromosome 13q12 that were highly linked to breast cancer in specific families[17]. The search for genes within these regions uncovered *BRCA1* and *BRCA2* on chromosomes 17 and 13, respectively[18].

Most cases of breast cancer occur sporadically in the absence of other affected family members, but because breast cancer is a common disease, approximately 20% of persons with breast cancer have a positive family history. Predisposition genes, including *BRCA1* and *BRCA2*, are relatively common. It is estimated that the frequency of carriers in the general population is between 1 in 800 and 1 in 400, with a significantly higher frequency in selected populations such as Ashkenazi Jews[19]. Approximately 1 in 200 women develops breast cancer due to the mutation of a high-risk gene, and such genes account for 5–10% of all breast and ovarian neoplasms. There are a variety of women who might consider genetic testing. These are summarized in Table 4. The potential benefits of having such genetic testing would include allowing the patient to plan medical care. This may also be useful for other family members who want to know the carrier's status and risks. It would allow unaffected family members to learn that they are not at increased risk or at lower risk than anticipated. It can alleviate the anxiety of 'not knowing' and hopefully thus improve family relationships. The drawbacks, however, can be significant. There can be heightened anxiety in carriers. It can interfere with family relationships and produce guilt in parents who transmit the gene. It can engender resentment in relatives, some of whom may be carriers and

Table 4 Potential candidates for genetic testing for hereditary breast and ovarian cancer

A woman under the age of 50 years who has a diagnosis of invasive breast carcinoma with or without a family history;

A woman who has a history of one or more affected first-degree relatives when at least one of the relatives was > 50 years old at the time of diagnosis;

A woman with a family history of male breast cancer;

A woman with a personal or family history of more than one primary tumor, e.g. bilateral breast cancer, breast and ovarian cancer;

A woman with breast cancer who has a relative with ovarian cancer or an aggregation of other cancers such as those of the colon, prostate or pancreas.

others not. Unfortunately, persons choosing testing, as well as known carriers, may encounter employer and insurance discrimination. The patient being tested may encounter uncertainty because of the unknown effects of surveillance and long-term results or capabilities of prevention.

Raloxifene

Like tamoxifen, raloxifene is also a selective estrogen receptor modulator. It is a benzothiophene derivative, unlike the triphenylethylene family from which tamoxifen is derived. Raloxifene, not unlike tamoxifen, was originally investigated as a treatment for advanced breast cancer. Preclinical studies indicated that raloxifene had an antiproliferative effect on both estrogen receptor-positive mammary tumors and estrogen receptor-positive human breast cancer cell lines[20]. In the 1980s, however, a small phase II trial revealed that raloxifene had no further antitumor effects in postmenopausal women with advanced breast cancer and in whom tamoxifen therapy had failed[21]. After information had surfaced about the neoplastic capabilities of tamoxifen on the uteri of postmenopausal women[22], there was renewed interest in raloxifene.

Raloxifene has selective estrogen receptor modulation (SERM)-like properties in that it has estrogen agonistic activity on bone remodelling and lipid metabolism. It was FDA approved for prevention of osteoporosis in postmenopausal women in December 1997. Its indication was extended to treatment of osteoporosis in October 1999. In terms of

raloxifene's effects on the endometrium of postmenopausal women, when compared with placebo[23], there were no differences in endometrial thickness, endoluminal masses, proliferation or hyperplasia. This corroborates previous information that raloxifene did not cause endometrial hyperplasia or cancer and was not associated with vaginal bleeding or increased endometrial thickness as measured by transvaginal ultrasound.

Preclinical data in animal models suggest that, like tamoxifen, raloxifene has potent antiestrogen effects on breast tissue[20]. The MORE trial involved 7705 postmenopausal women up to age 80 with established osteoporosis. In that trial, participants were randomized to receive raloxifene or placebo. Bone mineral density and fracture incidence were the primary study endpoints; breast cancer was a secondary endpoint. In the MORE trial at 4 years[24], raloxifene had significantly reduced the incidence of all invasive breast cancers by 72% compared with the placebo (RR 0.28; 95% CI 0.17–0.46). Raloxifene significantly reduced the incidence of invasive estrogen receptor-positive tumors by 84% compared with placebo (RR 0.16; 95% CI 0.09–0.30), but had no effect on estrogen receptor-negative tumors. The incidence of vaginal bleeding, breast pain and endometrial cancer in the raloxifene group was not significantly different from the placebo group. Similar to tamoxifen, thromboembolic disease including deep vein thrombosis and pulmonary embolism developed in 1.1% of women in the raloxifene group compared with 0.5% of women in the placebo group

($p = 0.003$). Currently there is no approved indication for use of raloxifene in the pre-menopausal woman. SERM compounds, structurally similar to clomiphene citrate, seem to have a different effect in pre- and postmenopausal women, as evidenced by the differences in the BCPT with tamoxifen in women < 50 and ≥ 50 years of age. Although there is no current indication for the use of raloxifene in premenopausal women, further study in such groups or with concomitant use of low-dose estrogen may be forthcoming.

Ongoing clinical trials

To compare the safety and efficacy of tamoxifen and raloxifene directly in reducing breast cancer risk among healthy women, the Study of Tamoxifen and Raloxifene (STAR) has been enrolling postmenopausal women who are 35 years or older and at increased risk for developing breast cancer. This study, which began in 1999 and is expected to run for at least 7 years, seeks to enrol 22 000 participants in a randomized double-blind fashion. Participants receive raloxifene 60 mg/day or tamoxifen 20 mg/day.

Raloxifene Use and The Heart (RUTH) is a double-blind placebo-controlled trial of 60 mg raloxifene that will include 10 000 women. Primary study endpoints are coronary disease and invasive breast cancer. Enrolment for this trial ended in August 2000, and study completion is estimated for 2006.

Aromatase inhibitors in breast cancer prevention

Substantial evidence supports the concept that estrogens facilitate the development of breast cancer in animals and in women, although the precise mechanism remains unknown[25]. The most commonly held theory is that estrogen stimulates proliferation of breast cells and thus statistically increases the chances for genetic mutation which could result in cancer. Aromatase inhibitors are a category of drugs that block peripheral conversion of androstenedione to estrogens. In pre-menopausal women, the primary site of this action is in the ovary. In postmenopausal women, this occurs predominantly in extra-ovarian sites including the adrenal glands, adipose tissue, liver, muscle and skin. Aromatase inhibitors might be more effective than SERMs in preventing breast cancer because of their dual role in blocking both initiation and promotion of breast cancer[26]. By inhibiting the initiation process these inhibitors would reduce the levels of the genotoxic metabolites of estradiol by lowering the estradiol concentration in tissue. At the same time aromatase inhibitors would inhibit the process of tumor promotion by lowering tissue levels of estradiol and thus blocking cell proliferation. However, because they are not selective, aromatase inhibitors would have an antiestrogen effect on bone and lipid metabolism, as well as inducing vasomotor symptoms.

Summary

Perimenopausal women are concerned about breast cancer. The incidence of breast cancer in premenopausal women seems to be rising at a rate faster than its proportion in the population. In perimenopausal women, estrogen levels increase prior to their ultimate decrease and absence[27]. Currently, tamoxifen is FDA approved for breast cancer risk reduction in high-risk women. The deleterious effects of tamoxifen in terms of uterine neoplasia and thromboembolic phenomena seem to be less relevant in women under 50 years of age. This has significant ramifications for the clinical care of the perimenopausal woman. Chemo-prevention for breast cancer risk reduction should be considered for perimenopausal women at sufficient risk. Definition of risk remains unclear. Hopefully future research will yield biomarkers that will be more clinically relevant for an individual patient than the currently employed combinations of population-based relative risks.

References

1. Bryant HU, Dere WH. Selective estrogen receptor modulators an alternative to hormone replacement therapy. *Proc Soc Exp Biol Med* 1998;217:45–52
2. Grady D, Gebretsakik T, Kerikowske K, *et al.* Hormone replacement therapy and endometrial cancer risk: a meta-analysis. *Obstet Gynecol* 1995;85:304–13
3. Miller BA, Fever EJ, Hankey BF. The significance of the rising incidence of breast cancer in the United States. In DeVita VT, Hellman S, Rosenberg SA, eds. *Important Advances in Oncology*. Philadelphia: Lippincott, 1994:193
4. Spicer DV, Pike MC. Risk factors in breast cancer. In Roses DF, ed. *Breast Cancer.* New York: Churchill Livingston, 1999
5. Bilimoria MM, Morrow M. The woman at increased risk for breast cancer: evaluation and management strategies. *CA Cancer J Clin* 1995;45:263–78
6. Gail MH, Brinton LA, Byar DP, *et al.* Projecting individualized probabilities of developing breast cancer for white females who are being examined annually. *J Natl Cancer Inst* 1989;81:1879–86
7. Ruffin MT, August DA, Kelloff GJ, Boone CW, Weber BL, Brenner DE. Selection criteria for breast cancer chemoprevention subjects. *J Cell Biochem* 1993;17G:234–41
8. Cummings SR, Duong T, Kenyon E, Cauley JA, Whitehead M, Krueger KA, for the Multiple Outcomes of Raloxifene Evaluation (MORE) Trial. Serum estradiol level and risk of breast cancer during treatment with raloxifene. *J Am Med Assoc* 2002;287:216–20
9. Jordan VC, Allen KE. Evaluation of the antitumor activity of the nonsteroidal antiestrogen monohydroxytamoxifen in the DMBA-induced rat mammary carcinoma model. *Eur J Cancer* 1980;16:239–51
10. Early Breast Cancer Trialists' Collaborative Group. Effects of tamoxifen and of cytotoxic therapy on mortality in early breast cancer: an overview of 61 randomized trials among 28,896 women. *N Engl J Med* 1988;319:1681–92
11. Early Breast Cancer Trialists' Collaborative Group. Tamoxifen for early breast cancer: an overview of the randomized trials. *Lancet* 1998;351:1451–67
12. Fisher B, Costantino JP, Wickerham DL, *et al.* Tamoxifen for prevention of breast cancer: report of the National Surgical Adjuvant Breast and Bowel Project P-1 study. *J Natl Cancer Inst* 1998;90:1371–88
13. Bur ME, Zimarowski MJ, Schnitt SJ, Baker S, Lew R. Estrogen receptor immunohistochemistry in carcinoma *in situ* of the breast. *Cancer* 1992;69:1174–81
14. Powles T, Eeles R, Ashley S, *et al.* Interim analysis of incidence of breast cancer in the Royal Marsden Hospital tamoxifen randomized chemoprevention trial. *Lancet* 1998;352:98–101
15. Veronesi U, Maisonneuve P, Costa A, *et al.* Prevention of breast cancer with tamoxifen: preliminary findings from the Italian randomized trial among hysterectomized women. Italian Prevention Study. *Lancet* 1998;352:93–7
16. Szabo CI, King MC. Inherited breast and ovarian cancer. *Hum Mol Genet* 1995;4:1811–17
17. Miki Y, Swensen J, Shattuck-Eidens D, *et al.* A strong candidate for the breast and ovarian cancer susceptibility gene BRCA1. *Science* 1994;266:66–71
18. Wooster R, Bignell G, Lancaster J, *et al.* Identification of the breast cancer susceptibility gene BRCA2. *Nature* 1995;378:789–92
19. Claus EB, Risch N, Thompson WD. Genetic analysis of breast cancer in the cancer and steroid hormone study. *Am J Hum Genet* 1991;48:232–42
20. Hol T, Cox MB, Bryant HU, Draper MW. Selective estrogen receptor modulators and postmenopausal women's health. *J Womens Health* 1997;6:523–31
21. Buzdar AU, Marcus C, Holmes F, Hug V, Hortobagyi G. Phase II evaluation of LY156758 in metastatic breast cancer. *Oncology* 1988;45:344–5
22. Neven P, Muylder X, Van Belle Y, Vanderick G, De Mylder E. Hysteroscopic follow-up during tamoxifen treatment. *Eur J Obstet Gynecol Reprod Biol* 1990;35:235–8
23. Goldstein SR, Scheele WH, Rajagopalan SK, Wilke JL, Walsh BW, Parsons AK. A 12-month comparative study of raloxifene, estrogen, and placebo on the postmenopausal endometrium. *Obstet Gynecol* 2000;95:95–103
24. Cauley JA, Norton L, Lippman ME, *et al.* Continued breast cancer risk reduction in postmenopausal women treated with raloxifene: 4-year results from the MORE trial. *Breast Cancer Res Treat* 2001;65:125–4
25. Santen RJ, Yue W, Nftolin F, Mor G, Berstein L. The potential of aromatase inhibitors in

breastcancer prevention. *Endocr Relat Cancer* 1999;6:235–43

26. Goss PE, Strasser K. Aromatase inhibitor in the treatment and prevention of breast cancer. *J Clin Oncol* 2001;19:881–94

27. Santoro N, Brown JR, Adel T, Skurnick JH. Characterization of reproductive hormonal dynamics in the perimenopause. *J Clin Endocrinol Metab* 1996;4:1495–501

Minimal access surgery for uterine disease

13

R. S. Neuwirth

Introduction

Minimal access surgery has become a driver of medical technology in the past 20 years. Endoscopes, catheters, balloons, stents, lasers, electrosurgery, sonography and angiography are but a partial list of the device explosion in cardiology, gynecology, obstetrics, orthopedics, and abdominal and chest surgery, to name a few of the disciplines affected. This chapter reviews minimal access techniques for non-malignant uterine conditions, but it does not address problems of pelvic floor herniation such as uterovaginal prolapse, rectocele, cystocele or urinary stress incontinence. It discusses functional disorders of the uterus in the perimenopausal patient, including problems caused by sex steroid hormonal production as well as problems related to sex hormone receptors. Bleeding due to anovulatory states is the most common problem, followed by the fibroid uterus, endometrial polyps and adenomyosis in the perimenopausal phase of life.

Anovulatory disorders are manifested by cycle disturbances and may be corrected by progestin pulsing or substitutional therapy with birth control pills, which suppress and replace disordered ovarian steroid production. The fibroid uterus is the second most common problem seen and is present in about 40% of women over the age of 40. It is primarily a disorder of hormone receptors in myometrial cell lines[1]. Fibroids can cause bleeding, which is typically progressively heavy and cyclical, but may be irregular as well. Women in this age group often have fibroids as well as episodes of anovulatory cycles, so the clinical picture may be mixed.

Furthermore, adenomyosis may be present and has been linked to an enlarged uterus, menorrhagia and pain.

The medical indications for treatment of menorrhagia, fibroids and/or adenomyosis are anemia and ureteral obstruction. Usually, the patient requests treatment for lifestyle problems of heavy and unpredictable menstrual flow, pelvic pain and pressure, or an abdominal mass. It is important to understand the patient's motives for seeking treatment in order to provide appropriate counselling as to risks, rewards and costs. The magnitude of the problems of perimenopausal bleeding, pain and a pelvic mass in perimenopausal women is large and has been the indication for well over half of the hysterectomies performed in the USA over the past century. From the epidemiological point of view, about 20% of all women undergo hysterectomy during their lifetime; about half of these are related to the perimenopausal problems discussed above[2].

History

Perimenopausal bleeding and pelvic masses are age-old problems. It was around the beginning of the 20th century that gynecologists began to treat the problem with hysterectomy, as anesthesia was becoming available and safer, and surgical techniques and instruments were being refined for abdominal and vaginal hysterectomy. Non-hysterectomy methods have been tried, including endometrial destruction by chemicals[3] and more recently by freezing[4], but these were too hazardous to be practical. During the next 75 years anesthesia techniques improved, blood and fluid management developed, antibiotic therapy for surgical infection was introduced and training programs in obstetrics and gynecology emphasized proper surgical training in hysterectomy technique. Morbidity and mortality rates from hysterectomy fell to current levels. Before the introduction of synthetic steroids in birth control pills, the practice was to perform curettage and then proceed with hysterectomy.

Transition to minimal access surgical options

After 1970 practices began to change because substitutional therapy for anovulation was a viable option for many patients. Furthermore, new diagnostic modalities appeared which enhanced the accuracy of the diagnosis of pelvic masses. Pelvic sonography and magnetic resonance imaging supplemented the classic bimanual examination. At the same time, laparoscopy and then hysteroscopy appeared, initially for diagnosis and later for surgical intervention. Ten years later, interventional angiography developed and shortly thereafter uterine artery embolization was introduced to treat uterine fibroids. As a result of this influx of new technology, a spectrum of treatment options has become available as alternatives to the classic abdominal and vaginal hysterectomy which were well established therapy by 1970. The pressure to explore these options by patients is understandably great. As minimal access procedures they appear attractive because they promise less pain and shorter recovery. Furthermore, women in the 21st century are usually in the work force in addition to having household and parenting responsibilities. Consequently, time is important to them. What is central to the decision-making process, beyond pain and recovery time, are the evidence-based data on effectiveness, cost and safety. The gold standard can be considered the classic

hysterectomy, as it is well known and is a cure for the problems. However, even hysterectomy has not been well defined in the long run, although the immediate and intermediate risks and benefits are well known (death rates and serious morbidity rates)[5]. Longer-term consequences of hysterectomy have not been well studied, although there are reports that the incidence of late bowel obstruction from adhesions may be 1.6% and higher[6]. There are reports suggesting that urinary problems and pelvic prolapse surgery are more frequent in women who have undergone hysterectomy for reasons other than problems of pelvic floor relaxation[7]. Sexual problems from lack of lubrication or a shortened vagina and psychological reactions to the loss of the uterus are at times reported by patients. The newer techniques must be verified as viable and safe clinical options for patients compared to the classic methods, as well as to each other, in order to provide patients with information that is understandable and reliable, so that they can make personal choices. While much solid information is not available, several techniques have undergone randomized prospective clinical trials as well as substantial clinical experience, but others have not. An overview is useful but is only a snapshot of a rapidly changing clinical database that will be evolving over the next few years.

Current options for interventional treatments for benign diseases of the uterus

Hysterectomy

The unique feature of hysterectomy is that it cures the problems of mass and bleeding and may relieve pelvic pain. It is probably the most expensive choice because of the operating time, surgical skills, hospitalization and recovery period. As the time-tested treatment, its death rate (approximately 0.1%) and major complications (approximately 8%) are standards against which minimal access techniques should be measured. Costs vary but $10 000 for the surgical and hospitalization costs are probably realistic in the USA. Less well documented are the indirect costs for recuperation and complications. As mentioned earlier, late postoperative bowel obstruction ranges from 1.6 to 3.0% from adhesions. Data suggest that the risk of a woman undergoing hysterectomy for reasons other than urinary stress incontinence or a form of pelvic prolapse may be doubled for subsequent surgery to correct some form of pelvic floor weakness.

Laparoscopic procedures

Since the introduction of laparoscopy in the late 1960s and the development of microchip television cameras, which transformed laparoscopic surgery into a team effort, a variety of laparoscopic procedures has been developed around hysterectomy. These include laparoscopically assisted vaginal hysterectomy, laparoscopic hysterectomy, plus operations similar in principle but with substantial technical differences. These procedures are more dependent on skill and instruments than classic abdominal or vaginal hysterectomy, and it is not clear that they are less costly than, or reduce immediate or long-term complications of, the standard hysterectomy procedures[8]. Hospitalization times may be shortened by these minimal access approaches but shortened hospitalization may also be related to patient motivation, case selection and technique, as reported[9] following vaginal hysterectomy. Complication rates from these procedures are difficult to ascertain but it is probable that they are not less than those associated with open procedures, and some may be higher, as they are more skill- and instrument-dependent. Case selection and surgical experience are major variables in success and complication rates. Certainly, laparoscopy has increased the use of vaginal hysterectomy in comparable cases, as it offers the advantages of abdominal control to the traditional restricted vaginal approach to remove the well-supported uterus of 12 weeks' size or less.

Another category of procedures performed is laparoscopic myomectomy or myolysis. The myomectomy is accomplished with mechanical devices and/or thermal energy instruments utilizing laser, electrosurgery or sonic power. Once excised the defect is closed with laparoscopically placed sutures and the mass removed with a morcellating device or via a culpotomy or minilaparotomy incision. Although hospitalization time is shorter, blood loss and operating time are difficult to compare unless a randomized prospective trial is organized against open myomectomy. Cohort studies do not provide a platform for evaluation of the technique versus the surgeon or the case selection.

Laparoscopic myolysis has been performed for several years[10]. Reports are scant but have indicated improvement in menorrhagia and reduction in uterine size. The technique employs electrosurgical needles to coagulate the blood supply at the base of the myomas and/or thermonecrose the mass. The myomas tend to shrink as the avascular necrosis proceeds, presumably replaced by scar. There have been unpublished reports about cases of infection and abscess but no database to estimate risk. There has been a report on pregnancy after myolysis[11]. The lack of data place this procedure in the category of clinical investigation.

Uterine artery embolization

Uterine artery embolization is a new addition to minimal access therapy for symptomatic benign conditions of the uterus[12]. It is performed under radiographic control by puncture of the femoral artery and catheterization of the uterine artery or its branches. Following angiographic identification, microspheres of variable sizes are injected to occlude flow to selected arterial branches. On occasion, ovarian artery branches are embolized if collateral circulation is present. The occlusion produces avascular necrosis of the distal tissues causing pain and then a gradual reduction in myoma size as well as reduction in bleeding. Complications have been reported including infection, target errors of the embolization, emergency hysterectomy and death[13]. Unfortunately, there are cohort studies and anecdotal reports, but very little long-term or comparative information. Very large fibroid uteri as well as cases with submucous myomas are apparently suboptimal for this technique. The method has been widely offered as a commercial treatment, but it is very difficult to counsel patients on success as well as risks. Costs of the procedure are about $2000 for the procedure plus the cost of overnight hospitalization. Data on recovery time, long-term success and long-term complications are limited[14]. There have been a few successful pregnancies after this procedure, but numbers are limited and many centers are wary of offering the procedure to women planning pregnancy.

Hysteroscopic procedures

Modern hysteroscopy was introduced in about 1970 following the solution of the problem of safe, controlled uterine distention using CO_2, 32% dextran 70 and dextrose in water. Operative procedures were reported soon thereafter, including septum repair, removal of polyps and removal of submucous myomas, particularly using the resectoscope, reported by Neuwirth in 1976[15]. The concept of hysteroscopic surgery was further advanced in 1981 by the report of Goldrath and colleagues of the technique of laser endometrial ablation[16]. DeCherney and Polan followed in 1983 with a report of resectoscopic endometrial ablation[17]. Thus, in a brief period, the transvaginal approach to perimenopausal bleeding and myomas was born. The laser and electrosurgical techniques were explored during this time but, owing to cost, complexity of equipment and skill dependency, the hysteroscopic electrosurgical techniques became the dominant hysteroscopic approach and were supported by instrument development, including continuous flow hysteroscopes, fluid balance systems and specialized electrodes to enable the surgery. Of particular importance was the finding that long-term

success in appropriately selected patients provided 90% of patients with clinical relief for 5–7 years and therefore often into the menopause[18]. Compared with hysterectomy, the procedure is brief, and had markedly lower mortality and morbidity risks. Furthermore, the lower cost and recovery time were attractive features[19]. The problems with the procedure were the specialized equipment and skills needed to perform the operations safely and effectively. These problems included mechanical and thermal uterine perforation as well as body fluid disturbances due to absorption of the uterine distending fluid during the course of the procedure, which could lead to congestive heart failure as well as hyponatremia with convulsions, coma and death[20]. The dilemma was the attractiveness of this palliative operation versus the low risk but very serious complications. Needless to say, many gynecologists were uncomfortable with this treatment, because of the high skill required to ensure safety, and have felt more comfortable to continue with the hysterectomy techniques they learned in training. In contrast to the other minimal access techniques, hysteroscopic endometrial ablation has had several databases collected on safety, as well as randomized prospective trials comparing safety, relief of symptoms and cost. In general these favor hysteroscopic endometrial ablation over hysterectomy for costs and safety, and are fairly comparable for relief of pelvic pain, patient satisfaction and return to an acceptable lifestyle[21]. In spite of these findings, recent reports from the UK indicate that the hysterectomy rate has not fallen, but the hysteroscopic endometrial ablation rate has risen to a plateau in the past several years[22]. The reasons for this are not clear, although several possibilities exist.

Non-hysteroscopic endometrial ablation

In spite of the reported advantages of hysteroscopic ablation, the technique has been mainly adopted by gynecological endoscopists and reproductive endocrinologists who focused enough time and effort to master the technique to achieve a high degree of safety and clinical success. Recognizing the advantages of endometrial ablation and the problems in incorporating it into regular clinical practice, Neuwirth and Bolduc designed[23] and tested[24] a non-hysteroscopic thermal balloon ablation device. US Food and Drug Administration (FDA) approval was granted in 1999 following a prospective, randomized clinical trial that showed therapeutic equivalence between the balloon ablation, Thermachoice® (Gynecare Inc., Somerville, NJ, USA), and rollerball hysteroscopic endometrial ablation in 12 centers in the USA and Canada[25]. It also showed fewer complications than the hysteroscopic technique in the hands of experts. Subsequent clinical use in over 100 000 cases has shown extraordinarily high safety, primarily because the heating system in the balloon shuts down if the pressure drops below 40 mmHg, which would occur if the balloon broke or if there were perforation into the peritoneal cavity. Thus, visceral injury is virtually precluded with this device.

A similar balloon device, Cavaterm® (Wallsten Medical SA, Norges, Switzerland), has been released in Europe and appears to have a parallel profile of safety and effectiveness[26]. It is reported to have 20 000 case experience. A circulating hot water system introduced by Goldrath, the Hydro-thermablator® (BEI Medical Systems, Peterboro, NJ, USA), has completed FDA trials and has received approval[27]. The system employs a hysteroscope with a special sheath through which hot saline at 80 °C is circulated through the uterus at approximately 300 ml/min. The treatment requires about 10 min. Safety from tubal spill or intravasation is based on an abort switch triggered by a loss of fluid from the system in excess of 10 ml. The method permits the gynecologist to view the endometrial cavity during treatment. Effectiveness is comparable to hysteroscopic rollerball ablation.

A cryotherapy probe has been presented to the FDA for blind cryoablation of the endometrium[28]. The technique requires repositioning and two freeze–thaw cycles. Localization is controlled by ultrasound and success rates vary fairly widely among the test sites. The numbers of cases are too small to define safety at this time. FDA approval for sale is pending.

A neodynium–YAG laser has been undergoing trials in Europe[29]. A special fiberoptic device, similar to an intrauterine device, is connected to the laser source by a fiberoptic connector cable. After proper insertion the device is activated for about 8 min and the laser light is guided in all directions in the endometrial cavity via the bundles in the device. Experience is limited but amenorrhea rates are said to be high. Considerations to ensure safety are unclear, other than that the laser energy does not penetrate more than 6 mm. Control of location of the device during activation is obviously very important.

Microwave endometrial ablation has been used in Europe for about 6 years. The microwave frequency is high, producing local but not deep tissue penetration. It consists of a probe with a microwave emitter at the top. The probe must be repositioned in the cavity to treat the entire cavity. It is rapid, requiring 2–4 min while intrauterine temperature is monitored. Control of placement is a problem, and intraperitoneal burn has been reported[30]. Success rates of 80% have been reported in early trials[31].

A bipolar electrosurgical ablation system consisting of an expandable metallic mesh, Novasure® (Novacept Inc., Palo Alto, CA, USA), has undergone testing for FDA approval[32]. The device is inserted blindly and location is checked by a gas pressure test. A vacuum is created to bring the endometrium into contact with the mesh electrodes. The treatment time is about 2 min. Complications have not been reported and the success rate in the early trials was about 80%.

A balloon device called Vestablate® (US Surgical Corp., Norwalk, CT, USA) was given an FDA trial and has been withdrawn[33]. The device is a balloon with electrosurgical plates on the surface which are designed to make close contact with the endometrial mucosa after inflation. The device apparently had good success rates but was withdrawn because the manufacture of the device at a commercial level was complex, primarily owing to the quality control of the number of sensor and power wires going to each electrode by which temperature and impedance were measured.

Summary

Minimal access surgery for uterine disease has undergone revolutionary changes in the past three decades. Classic surgical management was curettage and hysterectomy and this is still probably the dominant form of surgical management. Laparoscopic surgery bloomed after the introduction of the microchip videocamera and gave birth to laparoscopic hysterectomy, laparoscopically assisted vaginal hysterectomy, laparoscopic myomectomy, laparoscopic myolysis and other variations on the laparoscopic theme. Although the technology exists, case selection and endoscopic skills and judgement are considerations common to each of these therapeutic options. Cost comparisons are difficult to make, as are risk ratios, as objective information is difficult to obtain on complications. Skill is critical. Good, reliable and well maintained equipment is mandatory and long-term follow-up is essential. Although the procedures are attractive, because they promise smaller incisions as well as rapid discharge (key to the modern working woman), objective and comparative statistically valid data are not available.

The hysteroscopic approach also offers attractive options because there is no incision and menstrual control is often achieved. Again, endoscopic surgical skills, equipment, surgical judgement and case selection are important variables. Furthermore, hysteroscopic surgery is more unfamiliar to gynecologists trained in traditional programs where laparoscopic surgery is usually taught. Although comparative trials between hysterectomy and hysteroscopic endometrial ablation have shown lower costs and lower complication rates, longer-term comparisons are few. For example, endometrial cancer after ablation is only now

undergoing review. Late complications after hysterectomy such as intestinal obstruction and the risks of urogenital prolapse and stress incontinence have not been studied comprehensively in order to profile the consequences of the choice of surgery, i.e. hysterectomy or ablation. Furthermore, the flood of second-generation devices complicates matters, as each method needs a cost, success and risk profile. One advantage is that they are generally less skill dependent and therefore more easily studied for success, risk and cost.

Uterine artery embolization is a new approach which, at the moment, requires better definition of case selection, and more outcome data on success and safety. Immediate costs are available. One unique problem is that the treatment model has the radiologist performing the treatment and the gynecologist screening, counselling and carrying out post-treatment follow-up as well as acting as a surgical backup for surgical and medical complications. The interdependence creates a turf problem which has been resolved in many different ways in different settings and in many instances remains unresolved. It also tends to produce problems in collection of data on outcome.

Minimal invasive surgery for uterine disease has developed into a large spectrum of therapies. Comparative data on success, complications and costs are fairly comprehensive about some treatments and anecdotal about others. Certainly, hysterectomy is time-tested but, as mentioned, it too has data gaps now that comparisons are needed. Direct and indirect procedure costs and recovery costs can be estimated but may be illusory until long-term costs of failures and complications are factored in. Under the circumstances, safety should be the highest priority and should be compared to hysterectomy or hysteroscopic ablation, where the largest body of information on safety and effectiveness has been collected. As more experience develops with the new array of options now in early trial or clinical application, the factors for selection, failure and complications as well as a more global view of costs will emerge. Patient counselling and choice will then be less at the mercy of market forces. The good news is that technology is offering a variety of treatment options. The bad news is that a few thousand well-followed cases will be needed for each of the new techniques to be able to sort out the field and define the optimal minimal access choices for the many variations of uterine disease presented by the thousands of women who seek relief each year.

References

1. Wilson EA, Yang F, Rees ED. Estradiol and progesterone binding in uterine leiomyomata and in normal uterine tissues. *Obstet Gynecol* 1980;55:20–4

2. Carlson KJ, Nichols D, Schiff I. Indications for hysterectomy. *N Engl J Med* 1993;328:856–60

3. Salgado C. Esterellivacao provacado pela injeco intrauterine de caustico: document radiologicas. *Ann Brasil Ginecol* 1941;11:503

4. Drogemuller W. Effects of cryocoagulation of the endometrium. In Duncan G, Falb R, Speidel J, eds. *Female Sterilization*. New York: Academic Press, 1972:827–30

5. Thompson J. Leiomyomata and abdominal hysterectomy for benign disease. In TeLinde RW, Thompson JD, Rock JA, eds. *Operative Gynecology*, 7th edn. Philadelphia: Lippincott, 1992:676

6. Took AI, Platt S, Tulandi R. Adhesion related small bowel obstruction after gynecologic operations. *Am J Obstet Gynecol* 1999;180:313–15

7. Olsen A, Smith V, Bergstrom J, *et al*. Epidemiology of surgically managed pelvic organ prolapse and urinary incontinence. *Am J Obstet Gynecol* 1997;89:501–6

8. Munro M. Abnormal uterine bleeding: surgical management part III. *J Am Assoc Gynecol Laparosc* 2001;7:20–44

9. Stovall T, Summitt R, Bran D, Ling F. Outpatient vaginal surgery: a pilot study. *Obstet Gynecol* 1992;80:145–9

10. Goldfarb H. Nd : YAG laser laparoscopic coagulation of symptomatic myomas. *J Reprod Med* 1992;37:636–8

11. Vilos G, Daly L, Tse B. Pregnancy outcome after laparoscopic electromyolysis. *J Am Assoc Gynecol Laparosc* 1998;5:289–92

12. Ravina J, Bourat J, Fried D, *et al*. Value of preoperative embolization of uterine fibroma: report of a mullticenter series of 31 cases. *Contracept Fertil Sex* 1994;23:45–9

13. Vashecht A, Studd J, Carey A, *et al*. Fatal septicemia after fibroid embolization. *Lancet* 1999;354:307–8

14. Broder M, Landau W, Goodwin S, *et al*. An agenda for research into uterine artery embolization. Results of an expert panel conference. *J Vasc Intervent Radiol* 2000;11:509–15

15. Neuwirth R. A new technique for and additional experience with hysteroscopic resection of submucus fibroids. *Am J Obstet Gynecol* 1975; 131:91–9

16. Goldrath M, Fuller T, Segal S. Laser photovaporization of endometrium for the treatment of menorrhagia. *Am J Obstet Gynecol* 1981;140:14–19

17. DeCherney A, Polan M. Hysteroscopic management of intrauterine lesions and intractable uterine bleeding. *Obstet Gynecol* 1983;61:392–7

18. Derman S, Rehnstrom J, Neuwirth R. The long-term effectiveness of hysteroscopic treatment of menorrhagia and leiomyomas. *Obstet Gynecol* 1991;74:591–4

19. O'Connor H, Broadbent J, Magos A, McPherson K. Medical Research Council randomized trial of endometrial resection versus hysterectomy in management of menorrhagia. *Lancet* 1997;389:879–901

20. Overton C, Hargreaqves J, Maresh M. A national survey of the complications of endometrial destruction for menstrual disorders: the MISTLETOE study. Minimally invasive surgical techniques – laser, endothermal or endoresection. *Br J Obstet Gynaecol* 1997;102:1351–9

21. Crosignani P, Vercellini P, Apolona G, *et al*. Endometrial resection versus vaginal hysterectomy for menorrhagia. Long-term clinical and quality of life outcomes. *Am J Obstet Gynecol* 1997;1771:95–101

22. Bridgeman S, Dunn K. Has endometrial ablation replaced hysterectomy for the treatment of dysfunctional uterine bleeding? *Br J Obstet Gynaecol* 2000;107:531–4

23. Neuwirth R, Bolduc l. Intrauterine cauterizing method. *US Patent* 1992;5,105,808

24. Singer A, Almanza R, Gutierrez A, *et al*. Preliminary clinical experience with a thermal balloon endometrial method to treat menorrhagia. *Obstet Gynecol* 1994;83:732–4

25. Meyer W, Walsh B, Grainger D, *et al*. Thermal balloon and rollerball ablation to treat menorrhagia. A multicenter comparison. *Obstet Gynecol* 1998;92:98–103

26. Hawe J, Phillips A, Chien P, *et al*. Cavaterm thermal balloon ablation for the treatment of

menorrhagia. *Br J Obstet Gynaecol* 1999;106:
1143–8

27. Dobak J, Rybar E, Kovalch uk S. A new closed
loop cryosurgical device for endometrial ablation. *J Am Assoc Gynecol Laparosc* 2000;7:245–9

28. Das Dores G, Richart R, Nicolau S, *et al.*
Evaluation of Hydro-Thermablator for endometrial destruction in patients with menorrhagia. *J Am Assoc Gynecol Laparosc* 1999;6:275–8

29. Donnez J, Polet R, Rabinnivitz R, *et al.*
Endometrial laser intrauterine thermother-
apy: the first series of 100 patients observed
for one year. *Fertil Steril* 2000;74:791–6

30. Sharp N. Microwave endometrial ablation.
Presented at *A Consensus Meeting on Techniques
and Evidence in Endometrial Ablation*,
Middlesborough, UK, December 2000

31. Cooper K, Bain C, Parkin D. Comparison of
microwave endometrial ablation and transcervical resection of the endometrium for treatment of heavy menstrual loss. A randomized
trial. *Lancet* 1999;354:1859–63

32. Cooper J. Novasure bipolar electrosurgical
ablation system. Presented at *A Consensus
Meeting on Techniques and Evidence in
Endometrial Ablation*, Middlesborough, UK,
December 2000

33. Soderstrom R, Brooks P, Corson S, *et al.*
Endometrial ablation using a distensible mult-
electrode balloon. *J Am Assoc Gynecol Laparosc*
1996;3:403–7

Perimenopause: nutritional considerations

14

J. Lovejoy and M. Hamilton

Introduction

In examining the role of nutrition in the life of women who are progressing from premenopause to menopause, one must consider the nutritional challenges specific to the perimenopause as well as the impact of nutrition on the health of women throughout the lifespan. This chapter attempts to address these issues, despite sometimes inadequate data to answer many of the important nutritional questions that affect the lives of women during this period of transition.

Does nutrition affect the age of menopause?

Age of menopause appears to be strongly controlled by genetics, a major determinant being the age at which a woman's mother reached menopause[1]. Twin studies also suggest that 63% of the variance in age of menopause is due to genetic factors[2]. In addition to heredity, smoking is associated with a reduction in the age of menopause[3,4] and alcohol delays the age of menopause[5]. The first (tobacco use) should be avoided regardless of its effect on the age of menopause. The second (alcohol use), while of benefit in the prevention of cardiovascular disease[6], diabetes[7] and possibly osteoporosis[8,9], should be used in moderation, regardless of its effect on the age of menopause. Therefore, nutritional habits should be evaluated on their own merits, and not in terms of menopausal

age, since the elements of healthy nutrition are important to follow over the lifespan of women with the exception of certain areas that deserve special emphasis during the perimenopause and menopause. These will be addressed in later sections of this chapter.

Does age of menopause affect health? With respect to cardiovascular disease, there are data to support the notion that an earlier age at menopause increases the risk for cardiovascular disease and osteoporosis[10–14]. On the other hand, the risk of breast cancer increases with delayed menopause[15,16].

If age of menopause were important to manipulate by nutritional strategies, would we know how to influence the timing of this important transition? Little information exists concerning the effect of nutrition on the age of menopause. However, population data show that age at menopause varies between countries with widely different socioeconomic conditions and fertility rates. A recent international survey of age at menopause found that the age at menopause was lower in less developed compared to industrialized nations – for example, 44.6 years in Punjab, India versus 52 years in France – which may well reflect nutritional differences between these two countries[17]. The same study reported an inverse relationship between age at menopause and fertility rates, possibly due to the nutritional burden of multiple pregnancies, particularly in countries with more limited economic resources.

Does nutrition affect the symptoms of the perimenopause?

The symptoms of perimenopause are addressed in other chapters and include vaso-motor flashes, vaginal dryness, skin changes, and cognitive and mood changes. The accepted remedies for these symptoms include hormone replacement therapy in addition to a wide variety of untested comple-mentary methods, including herbal remedies, vitamins and other dietary supplements. The use of soy products has been studied with regard to reducing symptoms of hot flashes and improving cognition. The data on soy and hot flashes are largely equivocal, with most studies showing similar or only slightly greater symptom improvement with soy compared to control[18,19]. However, several randomized placebo-controlled clinical trials have found statistically significant improve-ments in hot flash frequency or severity during soy or isoflavone supplementation[20,21].

Few studies address the effect of soy con-sumption on cognitive performance. A recent study in rodents indicated that both estradiol and soy protein improved performance during a radial arm maze test which assesses working memory[22]. These researchers have also shown favorable changes in brain mark-ers associated with Alzheimer's disease in rats fed soy protein[23]. Clinical research addressing the effects of soy on human memory and cog-nition is lacking, and this is clearly an impor-tant area for future study.

Nutritional influences on health risk factors in the perimenopause

Many of the diseases commonly found in post-menopausal women, including osteoporosis, cancer, type 2 diabetes and cardiovascular disease, have their origins during the peri-menopausal period or even earlier in the life cycle. Furthermore, the majority of the chronic diseases seen in older women have a nutritional basis or component. Nutritional or lifestyle modifications during the perimenopausal

period may therefore have a significant impact on health during the postmenopausal years.

Obesity

Obesity plays a major role in a number of chronic diseases, including cardiovascular disease, type 2 diabetes and cancer[24]. The impact of the perimenopause on body com-position is discussed elsewhere in this volume. However, the importance of obesity as a nutri-tional concern in the perimenopause is so sig-nificant it must be mentioned here. Most studies have shown that menopause is associ-ated with a modest increase in body weight of approximately 1–2 kg. However, for some women, the weight gain is more substantial[25]. For example, in a longitudinal study by Wing and co-workers, the average weight gain in a group of 485 perimenopausal women was 2.25 kg, with 20% of the population gaining 4.5 kg or more[26].

Hormonal changes during the peri-menopause may influence cravings for high-sugar and/or high-fat foods and impact weight gain. In female rodents, high levels of estra-diol during the follicular phase of the men-strual cycle were associated with increased preference for sweet flavors and decreased appetite for fat, while during the luteal phase fat preference and intake increased[27,28]. In women, studies have similarly reported an increase in sweet preference in the follicular or periovulatory phases[29]. Ovariectomy increased food consumption in female rodents and monkeys, while a single injection of estradiol in ovariectomized female monkeys produced a significant decrease in food intake[27]. Because of the impact of hormones on food intake, maintaining appropriate caloric intake may be difficult for some women.

An additional factor impacting weight gain during the perimenopause is changes in lean body mass. Several studies have suggested that there are specific decreases in lean body mass in postmenopausal women[30]. Since decreases in lean mass are strongly associated with decreases in basal metabolic rate, these changes will lead to positive energy balance if not offset by decreases in food intake. Physical activity, specifically that targeted at maintaining muscle mass, is thus important to offset menopause-associated decreases in lean body mass.

Cardiovascular disease

Postmenopausal women are at greater risk for cardiovascular disease than are premenopausal women[31]. Much of the difference in cardiovascular risk in postmenopausal women is believed to be due to the loss of a protective effect of estrogen. However, nutritional factors also play a role.

The role of low-fat diets in preventing cardiovascular disease is controversial. While low-fat diets lower total and low-density lipoprotein (LDL) cholesterol, they have also been shown in some clinical studies to reduce high-density lipoprotein (HDL) cholesterol and increase triglycerides[32]. However, the majority of studies that have shown adverse effects of low-fat diets on serum lipids have controlled body weight. When body weight is allowed to fluctuate naturally, it tends to decrease slightly on low-fat diets[33]. Under these circumstances, we have recently shown that a low-fat diet fed for 9 months accompanied by weight loss did not result in decreased HDL cholesterol or increased triglycerides[34]. Similar findings were observed in the Dietary Approaches to Stop Hypertension (DASH) trial[35]. The DASH diet is a low-fat diet that is enriched in fruits, vegetables and calcium (mainly from low-fat dairy products). The DASH study demonstrated that low-fat, low-sodium, high-calcium diets improved blood pressure and also improved serum lipids[35,36].

Increased body weight *per se* has been shown to be an independent risk factor for dyslipidemia in the longitudinal Healthy Women Study[37]. In this study, women who gained weight during the perimenopause had a significant increase in serum cholesterol while those who maintained or lost body weight did not. Given the potential of low-fat diets to reduce calorie intake and assist in maintenance of a healthy body weight, their use in the perimenopause should be encouraged.

Soy protein, a natural source of phytoestrogens, has also been shown to have cardiovascular benefits. In a meta-analysis of controlled clinical trials[38], consumption of soy protein was shown to reduce total cholesterol by 23.3 mg/dl (9.3%), LDL cholesterol by 21.7 mg/dl (12.9%) and triglycerides by 13.3 mg/dl (10.5%) relative to consumption of casein. While the benefits of soy were greater in individuals with higher baseline levels of cholesterol, there were no differences in the effects by age or amount of soy protein consumed (31–47 g/day in the studies analyzed).

In addition to benefits on serum lipids and lipoproteins, phytoestrogens have also been shown to have beneficial effects on vascular reactivity. Impaired vascular reactivity has been associated with menopause and aging and can lead to hypertension and cardiovascular disease in older women. Nestel and colleagues[39] studied the vascular effects of soy isoflavones in perimenopausal and menopausal women not taking hormones. They observed that arterial compliance measured by ultrasound increased by 26% following 5–10 weeks of phytoestrogen supplementation. Animal studies suggest that soy protein consumption may be as effective as hormone replacement therapy in improving vascular reactivity. Clarkson and co-workers[40] studied coronary artery reactivity in ovariectomized female rhesus monkeys given conjugated equine estrogen (CEE), CEE plus medroxyprogesterone acetate, or soy protein. Monkeys fed soy protein had a 12% increase in coronary artery dilatation from control, compared with a 10% increase in monkeys receiving CEE and a 4% increase in monkeys receiving CEE plus progesterone. Thus, overall, consumption of soy protein appears to have substantial benefits for cardiovascular health and should be strongly encouraged in perimenopausal women.

The final nutritional consideration for perimenopausal women with regard to cardiovascular disease is alcohol intake. Moderate alcohol consumption has been shown to increase HDL cholesterol and lower LDL cholesterol in women[6] and is associated with reduced risk of coronary heart disease[41]. However, alcohol intake also contributes to excess calories and has been causally related to breast cancer (see below). Thus, no strong conclusion regarding alcohol intake in the perimenopause can be made. Women who currently consume alcoholic beverages in moderation can probably continue to do so and may reap some cardiovascular benefits, but there is no rationale for encouraging women who do not drink alcohol to start.

Type 2 diabetes

The prevalence of type 2 diabetes increases with age in both men and women[42]. However, several studies have suggested that menopause *per se* results in increased insulin resistance[43], a strong risk factor for type 2 diabetes. Menopause may therefore increase the risk for type 2 diabetes independently of the aging process.

Both insulin resistance and type 2 diabetes are strongly related to nutritional factors, including obesity. Obesity is a major nutrition-related risk factor for type 2 diabetes, with the majority of patients with diabetes being obese[44]. Obesity commonly results in insulin resistance, which may explain the close association between obesity and type 2 diabetes. Thus, avoiding excess weight gain during the perimenopausal and menopausal years is key to reducing diabetes risk.

Dietary fat intake also plays a role in the development of insulin resistance and type 2 diabetes[45]. Most studies[46,47], although not all, support a positive association between total fat intake and degree of insulin resistance in non-diabetic individuals. Additionally, several epidemiological studies have suggested that higher intakes of dietary fat predict the development of type 2 diabetes[48,49] and a recent study showed a positive association between total fat intake and hemoglobin A_{1c} levels in

men and women without diabetes[50]. The type of fat consumed is also important, with saturated and certain monounsaturated fats conveying a greater risk for insulin resistance and/or diabetes development than polyunsaturated fats[45]. Therefore, a low fat diet (particularly one low in saturated fats) is prudent for the perimenopause in terms of preventing diabetes, in addition to the considerations of heart disease and obesity mentioned above. Low-fat diets high in complex carbohydrates and fiber may further reduce diabetes risk, since low-fiber (high glycemic index) diets have been associated with increased diabetes risk[51].

Limited data suggest that soy protein may protect against the development of insulin resistance at menopause. Soy protein consumption results in a lowering of the insulin/glucagon ratio, primarily due to a decrease in fasting insulin[52]. In ovariectomized female monkeys, consumption of soy protein resulted in substantial increases in whole-body insulin sensitivity relative to casein consumption[53]. The effect of soy protein on insulin sensitivity and type 2 diabetes risk has not been studied in humans to our knowledge.

Finally, moderate alcohol consumption has been shown in epidemiological studies of both men[54] and women[7] to be associated with reduced risk of diabetes.

Osteoporosis

Postmenopausal osteoporosis and related hip and spine fracture are significant health risks in older women. In addition to the bone loss that occurs at menopause due to loss of estrogen, nutritional factors earlier in life are thought to play a major role in the likelihood of developing osteoporosis and fractures. Dietary calcium intake is clearly a major factor in both the development of peak bone mass early in life and also in protecting against bone loss after menopause. Women with low calcium intakes have lower bone density than those with high calcium intakes[55,56]. However, postmenopausal bone loss occurs despite normal–high calcium intakes. Supplementation with calcium and vitamin D has been shown to preserve and perhaps even increase bone mass in elderly women[57], while vitamin D alone has been shown to reduce hip fracture incidence in women living in northern climates where winter sun exposure is low[58].

Phosphorus, which is high in meat products and many carbonated soft drinks, causes calcium loss. A low calcium/phosphate ratio, typically caused by eating a preponderance of high-phosphorus foods, causes elevations in parathyroid hormone, resulting in calcium depletion from bone[59]. Furthermore, high-phosphorus, low-calcium diets are inversely associated with bone density in perimenopausal women, while calcium and phosphorus intakes independently do not predict bone density[60]. Therefore, in addition to increasing calcium intake, perimenopausal women should limit consumption of phosphoric acid-containing soft drinks.

High intakes of protein, particularly animal protein, increase urinary calcium losses[61] and cause bone loss in older women[62]. While there are some conflicting data on the effects of protein on bone loss, clearly excess protein intake (above the recommended daily levels) should be avoided and, when possible, preference should be given to consuming vegetable rather than animal protein.

Recently, there has been some indication that soy protein may be protective against bone loss[63]. Potter and colleagues[64] demonstrated that supplementing with soy isoflavones resulted in an increase in vertebral bone density relative to casein supplement over 24 weeks in postmenopausal women. Alekel and associates[65] similarly showed that consumption of soy protein isolate for 24 weeks attenuated bone loss in the lumbar spine of perimenopausal women. Researchers in Japan reported that dietary soy intake was associated with higher bone mineral density and lower bone resorption in postmenopausal women, and that soy had a stronger impact on these factors than energy, protein or calcium intakes[66].

Cancer

Cancer is also an age-associated chronic disease. Rates of cancer in women increase with increasing age, although the role of menopause *per se* in this increase may vary depending on the type of cancer. Many cancers are recognized as having a nutritional component; therefore, healthy diet changes during the perimenopause may help offset cancer risk in the postmenopausal years.

Obesity is a risk factor for both breast and endometrial cancer[67]. Furthermore, mortality from breast cancer is lower in postmenopausal women who are not obese[68]. Obesity also increases risk for colorectal cancer, which, although not specifically a 'women's cancer', is the second most common cancer in women after breast cancer[69].

The role of dietary fat intake in the development of breast cancer is controversial. Early epidemiological studies suggested a relationship between total fat intake[70], or intake of fried foods[71] and breast cancer. However, in general, more recent studies have not found an association between fat intake and breast cancer[72], although some studies report a relationship between either total fat intake[73,74] or saturated fat intake[75] and breast cancer. Associations between increased fat intake (particularly animal fat intake) and ovarian cancer[76] and endometrial cancer[77] have also been reported, although, as with breast cancer, these associations are not consistent across all studies.

Several studies have suggested that diets high in fruits and vegetables may protect against breast and other cancers[78]. This effect is likely to be due to the high concentrations of antioxidant vitamins and minerals (such as vitamins C and E, carotenoids and selenium) in fruits and vegetables. However, other phytonutrients and the fiber content of vegetables and fruits may also be important for cancer prevention. Additionally, since high-meat diets have been associated with breast cancer[79], it may be that vegetables and fruits reduce the risk by replacing meat and/or fat sources in the diet.

Soy protein consumption may be associated with reduced risk for certain cancers[80]. The incidence of breast cancer is significantly lower in countries where soy protein consumption is high, and in populations that consume more soy products[81]. In the USA, however, where soy consumption is generally low, there does not appear to be an association between phytoestrogen intake and breast cancer[82]. It is possible that higher intakes of soy are necessary to achieve a protective effect. Animal studies tend to confirm the beneficial effects of soy phytoestrogens on cancer risk. Genistein, an isoflavone in soy, decreased tumor volume and tumor blood vessel density in female nude mice injected with breast cancer cells, and increased breast tumor cell death in tissue culture in a dose-dependent manner[83]. Genistein has also been found to suppress estrogen-dependent tumor proliferation in vivo[84], although some studies have reported that certain doses of genistein stimulated tumor growth in vivo[85]. Because there are numerous other compounds in soy besides isoflavones which have anti-cancer effects (including Bowman–Birk inhibitor, inositol hexaphosphate, and β-sitosterol[86]), it may be that the adverse effects seen in some in vivo studies with high-dose, pure isoflavones would not occur if intact soy protein were used. More research is clearly needed to determine the exact effects of isoflavones in breast cancer.

Alcohol intake in women has been associated with an increased risk of breast cancer[87]. This increased risk is seen even in women who consume as little as 8 g of alcohol per day, who have a 50% increased risk of breast cancer[88]. This risk with alcohol intake is not seen for endometrial cancer[89] and even high levels of alcohol consumption are only modestly associated with the incidence of ovarian cancer[90]. Nevertheless, despite the potential benefits of moderate alcohol consumption on cardiovascular disease and diabetes risk, encouraging alcohol intake in perimenopausal women should be viewed with caution because of the reported increase in breast cancer risk.

General principles for maintaining health during and after the menopausal years

Weight control

As discussed above, average weight gain during the transition to menopause is modest, except for some women who experience more significant gains during this period. Because weight gain and obesity are associated with greater health risk the obvious message for perimenopausal women is that they should be aware of their weight and lifestyle factors that affect weight. This advice is reasonable, but may lead some to assume that the typical woman entering perimenopause is of normal weight. Increasingly, this is not the case. First, in both women and in men, weight increases with age until about the age of 60 years (Table 1). A 10-year longitudinal study of women aged 30–55 years revealed an average weight gain of 4.4 lb (2 kg)[91]. In this study, however, the incidence of major weight gain (i.e. more than 10 kg or 22 lb) was 12% in White women and 17% in African-American women. Specific to perimenopausal women, time trends show that the prevalence of body mass index (BMI) categories above 30 kg/m² in 40–49-year-old women and 50–59-year-old women has increased significantly since 1960 (Table 2), roughly a 60% increase in both age groups. Prevalence rates of overweight and obesity are significantly higher in low-income women and those belonging to minority groups, specifically African-American and Mexican-American women[92].

Therefore, in spite of evidence[93,94] that the healthiest BMI for middle-aged women is between 19 and 24 kg/m², significant numbers of women are entering menopause at weights that increase health risk. We also know from carefully conducted weight-loss trials that average weight loss is only in the range of 10–15% from initial weight. Thus, in practical terms, management of weight in perimenopausal women will involve two populations: one normal in weight (BMI less than 25 kg/m²) comprising 52% of the population

Table 1 Prevalence (%) of different body mass index (BMI) levels by age groups: USA, 1988–94. From reference 92

BMI (kg/m²)	Age (years)					
	20–29	30–39	40–49	50–59	60–69	70–79
25–29.9	18.5	21.2	25.9	28.8	34.2	32.8
30–34.9	8.6	14.1	15.5	20.2	17.4	15.9
35–39.9	4.3	7.3	6.5	9.6	8.7	5.2
> 40	1.8	4.4	5.0	5.7	3.7	3.9

Table 2 Prevalence (%) of obesity in women aged 40–49 and 50–59 years: USA, 1960–1994. From reference 92

BMI (kg/m²)	NHES (1960–62)	NHANES (1988–94)
Age 40–49 years		
> 30	17	27
30–34.9	11.6	15.5
35–39.9	3.7	6.5
> 40	1.7	5.0
Age 50–59 years		
> 30	20.4	35.5
30–34.9	14.0	20.2
35–39.9	4.4	9.6
> 40	2.0	5.7

NHES, National Health Examination Survey; NHANES, National Health and Nutrition Examination Survey

of women aged 40–49 and in whom we should encourage weight maintenance; and a second comprising 48% of the population, that is already overweight or obese and may not lose more than 5–15% from initial weight, even with the best weight-loss program.

In the overweight and obese group, but also in the normal weight group, the intensity of any therapeutic intervention will depend on the patient's and her family's history of risk factors, the longevity of family members, her body fat distribution and lifestyle, especially smoking and physical activity. Thus, there is greater concern about a woman with a BMI of 26 kg/m² and a waist circumference of close to 35 in (89 cm) (indicating a significant amount of visceral fat), who smokes, is sedentary and whose parents have diabetes and coronary heart disease, than a woman with a BMI of 32 kg/m², who does not smoke, is

physically active, whose parents lived into their eighties and nineties and who has a lower body distribution of fat[95,96]. One should also be aware that weight loss may decrease bone mineral density (BMD), but that this loss appears to be attenuated by physical activity[97]. Therefore, an assessment of osteoporosis risk is wise before initiating a weight-loss program so that preventive and monitoring measures can be planned.

Finally, because industrialized nations have attracted large numbers of immigrants from many parts of the world, Western nations are becoming multiethnic societies with demonstrated differences in health risk among women based on ethnicity[98–100]. Even in healthy African-Americans, Asians and Caucasians within given BMI ranges and age groups, there are differences in per cent body fat[101]. Not surprisingly then, it has been suggested that uniform standards for defining overweight, obesity and health risk may not be appropriate in view of these population differences[102]. The clinician must be aware that patients may have very different risks for the same BMI.

Having briefly described the complexity and number of variables associated with weight and health risk, it is important to return to a few basic principles that make intuitive sense. Those who are of normal weight should strive to maintain a normal weight and those who are overweight or obese should first of all gain no more weight, and preferably lose weight, with a goal of losing and maintaining a 10–15% loss from initial weight. This amount of weight loss, while less than most women hope for[103], has been shown to result in significant health benefits and, just as importantly, is a loss that is realistic and achievable[104,105]. The strategies by which these goals can be achieved are conceptually simple: controlling caloric intake and adopting a physically active lifestyle. These are briefly discussed in the sections that follow. However, for those who are unsuccessful in adopting healthier nutrition and physical activity habits, medications are available that can help patients to decrease caloric intake more effectively. Sibutramine is a centrally acting agent that increases satiety and reduces hunger. Orlistat is a lipase inhibitor that reduces the absorption of dietary fat. Medications are indicated only in those with a BMI greater than 30 kg/m², but may be prescribed in those with a BMI as low as 27 kg/m² if obesity co-morbidities that affect cardiovascular health or quality of life are present. Obesity surgery (gastric restriction or gastric bypass) is indicated in patients with a BMI of > 40 kg/m² or as low as 35 kg/m² in the presence of obesity co-morbidities. Surgery is the most effective treatment for patients with these levels of obesity and should be discussed as a possible option in appropriately selected patients. The indications for, and practical application of, the above therapies, medications and surgery, have been described[106].

Diet

The elements of a healthy diet in perimenopausal women are essentially the same as for women of all ages, with the exception that the previously discussed health problems and their prevention take on greater immediacy because of the impact of advancing age and the physiological changes associated with the approaching menopause. Therefore, the prevention and control of the dysmetabolic syndrome (Table 3), coronary heart disease and osteoporosis assume greater importance to women in their forties, especially those with a family history of these problems. A summary of nutritional factors affecting health risks relevant to perimenopausal women is shown in Table 4.

The rationale for adopting a diet that is low in saturated fat and simple sugars, is high in unrefined, complex carbohydrates and includes generous amounts of vegetables and fruits has been presented in an earlier section of this chapter. Essentially, the food pyramid describes what we believe to be the healthiest diet, but with these modifications: the base of the pyramid should strongly emphasize that unrefined complex carbohydrates are preferred, and that vegetable sources of protein,

Table 3 Components of the new ICD code for the dysmetabolic syndrome X (ICD 277.70–277.79)

Insulin resistance (denoted by hyperinsulinemia relative to glucose levels)
Acanthosis nigricans
Central obesity (waist circumference > 102 cm for men and > 88 cm for women)
Dyslipidemia (HDL cholesterol < 45 mg/dl for women, HDL cholesterol < 35 mg/dl for men, triglycerides >150 mg/dl)
Hypertension
Impaired fasting glucose or type 2 diabetes
Hyperuricemia
Hypercoagulability
Polycystic ovary syndrome
Vascular endothelial dysfunction
Microalbuminuria
Coronary heart disease

particularly soy, offer an advantage over animal sources of protein. Calcium from natural sources should be a major component of the diet in women of all ages but particularly so for women nearing the perimenopause and especially if there are risk factors for osteoporosis. A calcium supplement may be needed to achieve an intake of at least 1200–1500 mg daily. Some authorities recommend a multivitamin daily, even for those whose diet is varied and well balanced[107].

Because so many women are concerned about gaining weight during menopause, and because almost half of all women who enter the perimenopause are either overweight or obese, it may be useful briefly to mention a few basics concerning nutrition and weight control.

(1) In order to maintain weight one must consume no more calories than are expended throughout the day. To lose weight one must consume fewer calories than are expended during the day. Estimating caloric requirements, i.e. total daily caloric expenditure, is therefore important. It is difficult accurately to estimate an individual's daily energy requirement without sophisticated testing procedures, but one can obtain a rough

Table 4 Nutritional factors associated with improvement in specific health risks in perimenopausal women

Health condition	Nutritional recommendations
Obesity	low-fat/moderate-calorie diet, exercise
Cardiovascular disease	low-saturated-fat diet high in fruits, vegetables and low-fat dairy products; soy protein; maintain healthy weight; exercise; moderate alcohol intake
Type 2 diabetes	maintain healthy body weight; low-fat/high-fiber diet; soy protein; exercise; moderate alcohol intake
Osteoporosis	increase calcium and vitamin D intake; decrease phosphorus intake; select more vegetable (soy) rather than animal sources of protein
Cancer	high fruit and vegetable intake; low-fat intakes; maintain healthy body weight; soy protein; avoid alcohol to decrease risk of breast cancer

estimate by multiplying a person's weight in pounds by 10 kcal/lb, although this estimate will be inappropriately low for someone who is of normal weight or relatively muscular and lean. Alternatively, one can estimate metabolic rate from the revised WHO equations (Table 5). To maintain weight, then, one must eat approximately the same number of calories as the estimated daily requirement. To lose weight, one must consume less.

(2) Caloric restriction should generally not exceed 500–1000 below estimated daily requirements. Obviously, a well-balanced and varied diet will be the healthiest. On a reduced-calorie diet it is prudent to take a multivitamin as well as a calcium supplement, since some nutritional requirements may not be met when food intake is decreased, even with the most careful dietary plans. As mentioned, weight loss can lead to a decrease in BMD. Although obesity decreases the risk of osteoporosis, potential loss of BMD must be weighed against the benefits of weight loss. Again, physical activity attenuates the loss of BMD with weight loss[97].

(3) Studies have shown that meal replacements can also be effective, both for acute weight loss and for weight maintenance. One study[108] showed that replacing two meals and two snacks daily with a commercially available liquid meal and snack bar for an initial 3 months, followed by a 24-month maintenance phase using replacements for just one meal and one snack daily resulted in the maintenance of an 11.3% loss from initial weight, compared with a 5.9% loss in the control group assigned to conventional meals.

(4) Although high-fat, low-carbohydrate diets have enjoyed renewed favor in the past several years, there is no consistent evidence that the proportion of macronutrients in the diet makes any difference with respect to weight maintenance or loss[109]. A 1000-kcal diet consisting of olive oil (roughly 9 tablespoons) should result in about the same weight loss as a 1000-kcal rice diet (between six and seven cups of cooked rice). However, many patients who do go on low-carbohydrate, higher-fat and -protein diets, report dramatic weight losses, at least initially. Such losses can probably be attributed to a substantial decrease in caloric intake[110] resulting from the elimination of carbohydrates, which normally comprise 50% of caloric intake, as well as the satiating effect of animal protein, which is generally allowed in liberal amounts on these diets. The long-term health effects of low-carbohydrate, higher-fat diets are of concern with respect to cardiovascular risk. However, as mentioned, it is important to be aware that controversy continues to surround the issue of high- versus low-carbohydrate diets. There is evidence showing that low-fat, high-carbohydrate diets increase triglycerides and reduce HDL levels[111],

Table 5 Estimating energy needs. Revised WHO equations for estimating basal metabolic rate (BMR)

Men
18–30 years, BMR = (0.0630 × weight (kg) + 2.8957) × 240 kcal/day
31–60 years, BMR = (0.04984 × weight (kg) + 3.6534) × 240 kcal/day
Women
18–30 years, BMR = (0.0621 × weight (kg) + 2.0357) × 240 kcal/day
31–60 years, BMR = (0.0342 × weight (kg) + 3.5377) × 240 kcal/day

Estimated total energy expenditure = BMR × activity factor

Activity level
Low (sedentary); activity factor = 1.3
Intermediate (some regular exercise); activity factor = 1.5
High (regular activity or demanding job); activity factor = 1.7

particularly in patients who are insulin resistant and neither gaining nor losing weight[112]. A reasonable course to suggest is that a low-fat diet rich in complex carbohydrates is appropriate during weight loss[34], but that during weight maintenance it may be preferable to follow the generally recommended 30% fat diet, low in saturated fats with a relative increase in monounsaturated fats, along with a liberal intake of unrefined complex carbohydrates and fiber in the form of whole grains, vegetables and fruits.

(5) Lifestyles have changed for many working families who increasingly depend on foods prepared outside the home. Statistics from the US Department of Labor Bureau of Labor Statistics show that the food budget spent on eating out increased from 27% to 38% between 1974 and 1994[113]. In this study, compared with those who ate out less than five times per week, those who ate out 6–13 times per week ate more calories (2057 kcal versus 1769 kcal), more fat (80 g versus 61 g) but only slightly more carbohydrate and protein. From a practical standpoint, how often people eat out may not change, but education concerning healthier selections, in the choice of both restaurants and menu items, may help people limit the damage from the large portions and energy-dense selections that restaurants offer.

Physical activity

The health benefits of physical activity are well known in terms of cardiovascular risk[114–116] and diabetes[7]. In women, physical activity assumes even greater importance with increasing age, because of the increased risk of cardiovascular disease and osteoporosis associated with menopause.

While diet is a critical component of any weight-loss effort or of weight maintenance, the increasing prevalence of overweight and obesity in the USA and other industrialized nations over the past 50–100 years cannot be attributed to a major increase in food intake in the average person, since caloric intake from 1965 to 1995 has, on average, changed very little[117]. Clearly, those who fall in the higher BMI categories (Table 1) must consume a greater number of calories than those in the lower BMI categories, but perhaps not that many more. For example, a 40-year-old woman who is sedentary and weighs 300 lb requires a caloric intake of approximately 2600 kcal each day in order to maintain a stable weight based on the WHO formula to estimate daily caloric expenditure. A woman who weighs 150 lb requires less but not a great deal less, approximately 1850 kcal, a difference in food intake equivalent to a quarter-pound burger, small fries and a soft drink.

Many experts believe that the increasing prevalence of overweight and obesity is instead due to a decrease in physical activity over the past decades. The magnitude of the decline in physical activity is difficult to document, but James has estimated that, in Britain since 1970, daily energy expenditure from physical activity has fallen by 800 kcal[118]. Anyone over the age of 30 can probably recall several activities of daily life that require less effort to accomplish today compared with childhood days. For example, 50 years ago, when women were generally responsible for maintaining the home, washing was done by hand with a washing board, clothes were twisted until nearly dry, and finally carried to the clothesline to be hung. These are all fairly strenuous tasks, estimated to require an energy expenditure of 1500 kcal for a week's worth of household clothes[119]. Today, washing the same amount with a washer and dryer probably requires an energy expenditure of no more than 270 kcal. Considering that spontaneous physical activity, also called 'non-exercise activity thermogenesis' or NEAT ('fidgeting' in lay terms), can burn as much as 241–453 kcal in a day (somewhat less in women)[120] it is not surprising that the adoption of labor-saving devices has had an impact on energy expenditure and weight over the past several decades.

Therefore, the adoption of a program of physical activity that involves not just formal exercise but also an effort to increase the amount of energy expended in the activities of daily life (such as walking, climbing stairs, carrying one's bags and, in general, refusing the physical assistance of others to do things one can do for oneself), can do much to recapture the opportunities for physical activity that were taken from us by the invention and widespread use of labor-saving devices.

Physical activity increases caloric expenditure and minimizes the loss of lean tissue that normally occurs with weight loss (the tissue composition of weight loss or gain resulting from changes in food intake is about 75% fat and 25% lean tissue). While physical activity alone has only a modest impact on weight loss, physical activity appears to be essential in maintaining weight loss[121]. Even repeated small amounts of physical activity have an effect on energy expenditure; studies have

shown that the benefits of exercise can be attained in shorter segments, e.g. exercising three times per day in 10-min sessions instead of exercising 30 min once per day[122]. Therefore, the exercise prescription can be adapted to the patient's lifestyle and level of conditioning[123].

Aerobic activities will have the greatest impact on cardiovascular health, but in terms of weight loss, the total calories expended determine the effect on weight. Physical activities carried out with less intensity over a longer period of time will burn approximately the same number of calories as the same activity at a higher intensity over a shorter period of time. Walking 1 mile, for example, will burn approximately the same number of calories as jogging 1 mile (about 100 kcal depending on body weight).

Resistance exercises build lean tissues and can help attenuate the normal loss of lean tissue that occurs with weight loss. For those over the age of 50, resistance training can help to maintain lean body mass, which normally decreases after that age[30]. Resistance training has special benefits in terms of quality of life to people over 60 years who are generally less interested in running a marathon than continuing to enjoy the activities of daily life, i.e. having the strength and flexibility to climb stairs, shop, step out of a shower without falling and travel to visit friends and family, whether far or near. Resistance exercises also reduce the risk of osteoporosis, as do impact exercises.

Nevertheless, from a behavioral viewpoint the specific type of physical activity is less important than settling on an activity the patient enjoys and will do on a consistent basis.

Since gaining no more weight is possibly the most important goal for all women, whether normal weight or overweight, it is instructive to review the experience of persons in the National Weight Control Registry who have lost weight and maintained their loss for a significant period of time[121]. In a study of 3000 subjects who have maintained an average weight loss of 66 lb for over 5 years, the major ingredients of success were: following a diet low in fat (24% of total calories from fat);

self-monitoring of body weight (daily) and food intake; and consistent physical activity. Of interest, the level of physical activity reported was considerably higher than the 30 min a day recommended to the general public. Women reported expending 2545 kcal per week in physical activity (equivalent to walking about 25 miles) and men, 3293 kcal per week. Walking was an important physical activity in over 75% of subjects. Twenty-four per cent of men and 20% of women reported weight lifting. Subjects reported that considerable effort was required to maintain weight loss, but that after 2 years of maintenance, these efforts seemed easier to sustain. Of interest, almost half reported being overweight children and 46% reported having one obese parent and 26% having two obese parents.

Finally, physical activity, as reflected by fitness level, may be related to better adherence to a healthy diet[124]. In this study, fitness in women was associated with reduced intake of saturated fat, and increased consumption of dietary fiber, minerals and vitamins.

Stress

Stress is part of the human condition and can affect behavior in many ways, but perhaps most seductively with respect to food intake and physical activity. Every clinician knows, either through personal experience or through his or her patients, that the best-intentioned nutrition and physical activity plans often fail in the face of a stressful event, no matter how seemingly minor. It is intuitively apparent that the effect of stress on food intake, either an increase or a decrease, is due to emotional arousal and the relief afforded by eating, especially in those who overeat in response to stress. Studies indicate, however, that physiological and hormonal mechanisms also play an important role. Glucocorticoids have been associated with increased food intake[125] and clinicians are certainly familiar with the appetite-stimulating effects of steroid therapy. In a recent study of women aged 30–45 years, caloric intake was greatest in women who had the greatest increase in cortisol secretion (determined by salivary cortisol) in response to a standard mental stress compared with women who were low cortisol reactors in response to the same stressor[126]. On control days (days without an administered stress stimulus) high and low cortisol reactors ate approximately the same number of calories. High cortisol reactors ate more sweet foods on stress as well as control days. In another study of the effect of a mental stress on food intake, those whose response to stress was greatest (as determined by blood pressure, heart rate and mood) ate more sweet and high-fat foods[127]. Because so many women work outside the home today, the opportunities to experience stress resulting from the dual responsibilities at home and at work are greatly magnified. One study of workplace stress showed that periods of high stress, as defined by longer working hours, was associated with a higher intake of saturated fat and sugar. Furthermore, restrained eaters (those who habitually try to limit their food intake) were more likely to overeat in response to work stress[128].

The effect of stress on physical activity habits is also intuitively apparent. While some respond to stress by increasing their level of physical activity, it is probably more common that most will become less physically active during periods of stress, in spite of the fact that physical activity has been shown to reduce stress, and the risk of cardiovascular disease, diabetes and osteoporosis. Thus, stress can have a significant effect on behavior with respect to nutrition and physical activity. The issue of stress and health has an enormous literature, including sentinel work by Bjorntorp[129,130]. Managing stress is a more difficult issue and has become a huge industry in the USA, as evidenced by bookstores whose shelves are heavy with self-help books, weekend seminars on coping with just about every situation or condition of human existence, and counselling from a wide variety of well-trained and capable therapists. For some, these avenues are readily available, but for many women these resources are not accessible because of economic, social or cultural barriers. Nevertheless, providing referral to appropriate community resources when available, along with practical advice about nutrition and physical activity, sends a message: nutrition, physical activity and how one manages one's life are important to health and quality of life, and therefore worth talking about, even for a busy clinician.

References

1. Torgerson DJ, Thomas RE, Campbell MK, Reid DM. Alcohol consumption and age of maternal menopause are associated with menopause onset. *Maturitas* 1997;26:21–5

2. Snieder H, MacGregor AJ, Spector TD. Genes control the cessation of a woman's reproductive life: a twin study of hysterectomy and age at menopause. *J Clin Endocrinol Metab* 1998; 83:1875–80

3. Do KA, Treloar SA, Pandeya N, *et al*. Predictive factors of age at menopause in a large Australian twin study. *Hum Biol* 1998;70:1073–91

4. Willett W, Stampfer MJ, Bain C, *et al*. Cigarette smoking, relative weight, and menopause. *Am J Epidemiol* 1983;117:651–8

5. Torgerson DJ, Avenell A, Russell IT, Reid DM. Factors associated with onset of menopause in women aged 45–49. *Maturitas* 1994;19:83–92

6. van der Gaag MS, Sierksma A, Schaafsma G, *et al*. Moderate alcohol consumption and changes in postprandial lipoproteins of premenopausal and postmenopausal women: a diet-controlled, randomized intervention study. *J Womens Health Gend Based Med* 2000;9: 607–16

7. Hu FB, Manson JE, Stampfer MJ, *et al*. Diet, lifestyle, and the risk of type 2 diabetes mellitus in women. *N Engl J Med* 2001;345:790–7

8. Siris ES, Miller PD, Barrett-Connor E, *et al*. Identification and fracture outcomes of undiagnosed low bone mineral density in postmenopausal women: results from the National Osteoporosis Risk Assessment. *J Am Med Assoc* 2001;286:2815–22

9. Ganry O, Baudoin C, Fardellone P. Effect of alcohol intake on bone mineral density in elderly women: The EPIDOS Study. Epidemiologie de l'Osteoporose. *Am J Epidemiol* 2000; 151:773–80

10. van der Schouw YT, van der Graaf Y, Steyerberg EW, Eijkemans JC, Banga JD. Age at menopause as a risk factor for cardiovascular mortality. *Lancet* 1996;347:714–18

11. Jacobsen BK, Knutsen SF, Fraser GE. Age at natural menopause and total mortality and mortality from ischemic heart disease: the Adventist Health Study. *J Clin Epidemiol* 1999;52:303–7

12. Joakimsen O, Bonaa KH, Stensland-Bugge E, Jacobsen BK. Population-based study of age at menopause and ultrasound assessed carotid atherosclerosis: The Tromso Study. *J Clin Epidemiol* 2000;53:525–30

13. NIH Consensus Development Panel on Osteoporosis Prevention, Diagnosis, and Therapy. Osteoporosis prevention, diagnosis, and therapy. *J Am Med Assoc* 2001;285:785–95

14. Osei-Hyiaman D, Satoshi T, Ueji M, Hideto T, Kano K. Timing of menopause, reproductive years, and bone mineral density: a cross-sectional study of postmenopausal Japanese women. *Am J Epidemiol* 1998;148:1055–61

15. Sasco AJ. Epidemiology of breast cancer: an environmental disease? *Apmis* 2001;109:321–32

16. Claus EB, Stowe M, Carter D. Breast carcinoma *in situ*: risk factors and screening patterns. *J Natl Cancer Inst* 2001;93:1811–17

17. Thomas F, Renaud F, Benefice E, de Meeus T, Guegan JF. International variability of ages at menarche and menopause: patterns and main determinants. *Hum Biol* 2001;73:271–90

18. Quella SK, Loprinzi CL, Barton DL, *et al*, Evaluation of soy phytoestrogens for the treatment of hot flashes in breast cancer survivors: a North Central Cancer Treatment Group trial. *J Clin Oncol* 2000;18:1068–74

19. St Germain A, Peterson CT, Robinson JG, Alekel DL. Isoflavone-rich or isoflavone-poor soy protein does not reduce menopausal symptoms during 24 weeks of treatment. *Menopause* 2001;8:17–26

20. Washburn S, Burke GL, Morgan T, Anthony M. Effect of soy protein supplementation on serum lipoproteins, blood pressure, and menopausal symptoms in perimenopausal women. *Menopause* 1999;6:7–13

21. Upmalis DH, Lobo R, Bradley L, Warren M, Cone FL, Lamia CA. Vasomotor symptom relief by soy isoflavone extract tablets in postmenopausal women: a multicenter, double-blind, randomized, placebo-controlled study. *Menopause* 2000;7:236–42

22. Pan Y, Anthony M, Watson S, Clarkson TB. Soy phytoestrogens improve radial arm maze performance in ovariectomized retired breeder rats and do not attenuate benefits of

17beta-estradiol treatment. *Menopause* 2000;7: 230–5

23. Pan Y, Anthony M, Clarkson TB. Evidence for up-regulation of brain-derived neurotrophic factor mRNA by soy phytoestrogens in the frontal cortex of retired breeder female rats. *Neurosci Lett* 1999;261:17–20

24. National Institutes of Health. Clinical Guidelines on the Identification, Evaluation, and Treatment of Overweight and Obesity in Adults – The Evidence Report. *Obes Res* 1998;6(Suppl 2):51S–209S

25. Tchernof A, Poehlman ET. Effects of the menopause transition on body fatness and body fat distribution. *Obes Res* 1998;6:246–54

26. Wing RR, Matthews KA, Kuller LH, Meilahn EN, Plantinga PL. Weight gain at the time of menopause. *Arch Intern Med* 1991;151:97–102

27. Wade G. Sex hormones, regulatory behaviors, and body weight. *Adv Study Behav* 1976;6: 201–79

28. Geiselman PJ, Martin JR, Vanderweele DA, Novin D. Dietary self-selection in cycling and neonatally ovariectomized rats. *Appetite* 1981; 2:87–101

29. Wright P, Crow R. Menstrual cycle: effect on sweetness preferences in women. *Horm Behav* 1973;4:387

30. Douchi T, Yamamoto S, Nakamura S, *et al.* The effect of menopause on regional and total body lean mass. *Maturitas* 1998;29:247–52

31. Sullivan JM, Fowlkes LP. The clinical aspects of estrogen and the cardiovascular system. *Obstet Gynecol* 1996;87:36S–43S

32. Clarke R, Frost C, Collins R, Appleby P, Peto R. Dietary lipids and blood cholesterol: quantitative meta-analysis of metabolic ward studies. *Br Med J* 1997;314:112–17

33. Bray GA, Popkin BM. Dietary fat intake does affect obesity! *Am J Clin Nutr* 1998;68:1157–73

34. Lovejoy JC, Lefevre M, Bray GA, *et al.* Beneficial effect of a low-fat diet on health risk factors is mediated by weight-loss in middle age men. *Obes Res* 2000;8:56S

35. Appel LJ, Moore TJ, Obarzanek E, *et al.* A clinical trial of the effects of dietary patterns on blood pressure. DASH Collaborative Research Group. *N Engl J Med* 1997;336:1117–24

36. Obarzanek E, Sacks FM, Vollmer WM, *et al.* Effects on blood lipids of a blood pressure-lowering diet: the Dietary Approaches to Stop Hypertension (DASH) trial. *Am J Clin Nutr* 2001;74:80–9

37. Kuller LH, Simkin-Silverman LR, Wing RR, Meilahn EN, Ives DG. Women's Healthy Lifestyle Project: a randomized clinical trial: results at 54 months. *Circulation* 2001;103:32–7

38. Anderson JW, Johnstone BM, Cook-Newell ME. Meta-analysis of the effects of soy protein intake on serum lipids. *N Engl J Med* 1995; 333:276–82

39. Nestel PJ, Yamashita T, Sasahara T, *et al.* Soy isoflavones improve systemic arterial compliance but not plasma lipids in menopausal and perimenopausal women. *Arterioscler Thromb Vasc Biol* 1997;17:3392–8

40. Clarkson TB, Anthony MS, Williams JK, Honore EK, Cline JM. The potential of soybean phytoestrogens for postmenopausal hormone replacement therapy. *Proc Soc Exp Biol Med* 1998;217:365–8

41. Fuchs CS, Stampfer MJ, Colditz GA, *et al.* Alcohol consumption and mortality among women. *N Engl J Med* 1995;332:1245–50

42. National Diabetes Data Group. *Diabetes in America*. Washington, DC: National Institutes of Health, 1995:87–8

43. DeNino WF, Tchernof A, Dionne IJ, *et al.* Contribution of abdominal adiposity to age-related differences in insulin sensitivity and plasma lipids in healthy nonobese women. *Diabetes Care* 2001;24:925–32

44. Pi-Sunyer FX. Health implications of obesity. *Am J Clin Nutr* 1991;53:1595S–603S

45. Lovejoy JC. Dietary fatty acids and insulin resistance. *Curr Atheroscler Rep* 1999;1:215–20

46. Fukagawa NK, Anderson JW, Hageman G, Young VR, Minaker KL. High-carbohydrate, high-fiber diets increase peripheral insulin sensitivity in healthy young and old adults. *Am J Clin Nutr* 1990;52:524–8

47. Lovejoy JC, Windhauser MM, Rood JC, de la Bretonne JA. Effect of a controlled high-fat versus low-fat diet on insulin sensitivity and leptin levels in African-American and Caucasian women. *Metabolism* 1998;47:1520–4

48. Feskens EJ, Virtanen SM, Rasanen L, *et al.* Dietary factors determining diabetes and impaired glucose tolerance. A 20-year follow-up of the Finnish and Dutch cohorts of the Seven Countries Study. *Diabetes Care* 1995;18: 1104–12

49. Mayer-Davis EJ, Monaco JH, Hoen HM, *et al.* Dietary fat and insulin sensitivity in a triethnic population: the role of obesity. The Insulin Resistance Atherosclerosis Study (IRAS). *Am J Clin Nutr* 1997;65:79–87

50. Harding AH, Sargeant LA, Welch A, *et al.* Fat consumption and HbA(1c) levels: the EPIC-Norfolk study. *Diabetes Care* 2001;24:1911–16

51. Salmeron J, Manson JE, Stampfer MJ, Colditz GA, Wing AL, Willett WC. Dietary fiber, glycemic load, and risk of non-insulin-dependent diabetes mellitus in women. *J Am Med Assoc* 1997;277:472–7

52. Sanchez A, Hubbard RW. Plasma amino acids and the insulin/glucagon ratio as an explanation for the dietary protein modulation

of atherosclerosis. *Med Hypotheses* 1991; 36:27–32

53. Wagner JD, Cefalu WT, Anthony MS, Litwak KN, Zhang L, Clarkson TB. Dietary soy protein and estrogen replacement therapy improve cardio-vascular risk factors and decrease aortic choles-teryl ester content in ovariectomized cynomolgus monkeys. *Metabolism* 1997;46:698–705

54. Wei M, Gibbons LW, Mitchell TL, Kampert JB, Blair SN. Alcohol intake and incidence of type 2 diabetes in men. *Diabetes Care* 2000;23:18–22

55. Reed JA, Anderson JJ, Tylavsky FA, Gallagher PN Jr. Comparative changes in radial-bone density of elderly female lacto-ovovegetarians and omnivores. *Am J Clin Nutr* 1994;59: 1197S–202S

56. Riggs BL, O'Fallon WM, Muhs J, O'Connor MK, Kumar R, Melton LJ 3rd. Long-term effects of calcium supplementation on serum parathyroid hormone level, bone turnover, and bone loss in elderly women. *J Bone Miner Res* 1998;13:168–74

57. Chapuy MC, Arlot ME, Duboeuf F, *et al.* Vitamin D3 and calcium to prevent hip frac-tures in the elderly women. *N Engl J Med* 1992;327:1637–42

58. Heikinheimo RJ, Inkovaara JA, Harju EJ, *et al.* Annual injection of vitamin D and fractures of aged bones. *Calcif Tissue Int* 1992;51:105–10

59. Calvo MS, Kumar R, Heath H. Persistently ele-vated parathyroid hormone secretion and action in young women after four weeks of ingesting high phosphorus, low calcium diets. *J Clin Endocrinol Metab* 1990;70:1334–40

60. Brot C, Jorgensen N, Madsen OR, Jensen LB, Sorensen OH. Relationships between bone mineral density, serum vitamin D metabolites and calcium : phosphorus intake in healthy perimenopausal women. *J Intern Med* 1999; 245:509–16

61. Kerstetter JE, Allen LH. Dietary protein increases urinary calcium. *J Nutr* 1990;120: 134–6

62. Sellmeyer DE, Stone KL, Sebastian A, Cummings SR. A high ratio of dietary animal to vegetable protein increases the rate of bone loss and the risk of fracture in postmenopausal women. Study of Osteoporotic Fractures Research Group. *Am J Clin Nutr* 2001;73:118–22

63. Scheiber MD, Rebar RW. Isoflavones and post-menopausal bone health: a viable alternative to estrogen therapy? *Menopause* 1999;6:233–41

64. Potter SM, Baum JA, Teng H, Stillman RJ, Shay NF, Erdman JW Jr. Soy protein and isoflavones: their effects on blood lipids and bone density in postmenopausal women. *Am J Clin Nutr* 1998;68:1375S–9S

65. Alekel DL, Germain AS, Peterson CT, Hanson KB, Stewart JW, Toda T. Isoflavone-rich soy protein isolate attenuates bone loss in the lumbar spine of perimenopausal women. *Am J Clin Nutr* 2000;72:844–52

66. Horiuchi T, Onouchi T, Takahashi M, Ito H, Orimo H. Effect of soy protein on bone meta-bolism in postmenopausal Japanese women. *Osteoporos Int* 2000;11:721–4

67. Schindler AE. Obesity and cancer risk in women. *Arch Gynecol Obstet* 1997;261:21–4

68. Zhang S, Folsom AR, Sellers TA, Kushi LH, Potter JD. Better breast cancer survival for postmenopausal women who are less over-weight and eat less fat. The Iowa Women's Health Study. *Cancer* 1995;76:275–83

69. Slattery ML, Potter J, Caan B, *et al.* Energy balance and colon cancer – beyond physical activity. *Cancer Res* 1997;57:75–80

70. Phillips RL. Role of life-style and dietary habits in risk of cancer among Seventh-day Adventists. *Cancer Res* 1975;35:3513–22

71. Miller AB, Kelly A, Choi NW, *et al.* A study of diet and breast cancer. *Am J Epidemiol* 1978; 107:499–509

72. Lee MM, Lin SS. Dietary fat and breast cancer. *Annu Rev Nutr* 2000;20:221–48

73. Kushi LH, Sellers TA, Potter JD, *et al.* Dietary fat and postmenopausal breast cancer. *J Natl Cancer Inst* 1992;84:1092–9

74. Barrett-Connor E, Friedlander NJ. Dietary fat, calories, and the risk of breast cancer in postmenopausal women: a prospective popu-lation-based study. *J Am Coll Nutr* 1993;12: 390–9

75. Smith-Warner SA, Spiegelman D, Adami HO, *et al.* Types of dietary fat and breast cancer: a pooled analysis of cohort studies. *Int J Cancer* 2001;92:767–74

76. Cramer DW, Welch WR, Hutchison GB, Willett W, Scully RE. Dietary animal fat in relation to ovarian cancer risk. *Obstet Gynecol* 1984;63: 833–8

77. Potischman N, Swanson CA, Brinton LA, *et al.* Dietary associations in a case–control study of endometrial cancer. *Cancer Causes Control* 1993;4:239–50

78. Gandini S, Merzenich H, Robertson C, Boyle P. Meta-analysis of studies on breast cancer risk and diet: the role of fruit and vegetable consumption and the intake of associated micronutrients. *Eur J Cancer* 2000;36:636–46

79. Bingham SA. High-meat diets and cancer risk. *Proc Nutr Soc* 1999;58:243–8

80. Messina MJ, Persky V, Setchell KD, Barnes S. Soy intake and cancer risk: a review of the *in vitro* and *in vivo* data. *Nutr Cancer* 1994;21: 113–31

81. Wu AH, Ziegler RG, Horn-Ross PL, *et al.* Tofu and risk of breast cancer in Asian-Americans. *Cancer Epidemiol Biomarkers Prev* 1996;5:901–6

82. Horn-Ross PL, John EM, Lee M, *et al.* Phytoestrogen consumption and breast cancer risk in a multiethnic population: the Bay Area Breast Cancer Study. *Am J Epidemiol* 2001;154: 434–41

83. Shao ZM, Wu J, Shen ZZ, Barsky SH. Genistein exerts multiple suppressive effects on human breast carcinoma cells. *Cancer Res* 1998;58:4851–7

84. Constantinou AI, Krygier AE, Mehta RR. Genistein induces maturation of cultured human breast cancer cells and prevents tumor growth in nude mice. *Am J Clin Nutr* 1998;68: 1426S–30S

85. Allred CD, Allred KF, Ju YH, Virant SM, Helferich WG. Soy diets containing varying amounts of genistein stimulate growth of estrogen-dependent (MCF-7) tumors in a dose-dependent manner. *Cancer Res* 2001;61: 5045–50

86. Kennedy AR. The evidence for soybean products as cancer preventive agents. *J Nutr* 1995;125:733S–43S

87. Longnecker MP. Alcoholic beverage consumption in relation to risk of breast cancer: meta-analysis and review. *Cancer Causes Control* 1994;5:73–82

88. Martin-Moreno JM, Boyle P, Gorgojo L, *et al.* Alcoholic beverage consumption and risk of breast cancer in Spain. *Cancer Causes Control* 1993;4:345–53

89. Gapstur SM, Potter JD, Sellers TA, Kushi LH, Folsom AR. Alcohol consumption and post-menopausal endometrial cancer: results from the Iowa Women's Health Study. *Cancer Causes Control* 1993;4:323–9

90. La Vecchia C, Negri E, Franceschi S, Parazzini F, Gentile A, Fasoli M. Alcohol and epithelial ovarian cancer. *J Clin Epidemiol* 1992;45:1025–30

91. Williamson DF, Kahn HS, Byers T. The 10-y incidence of obesity and major weight gain in black and white US women aged 30–55 y. *Am J Clin Nutr* 1991;53:1515S–18S

92. Flegal KM, Carroll MD, Kuczmarski RJ, Johnson CL. Overweight and obesity in the United States: prevalence and trends, 1960–1994. *Int J Obes Relat Metab Disord* 1998;22:39–47

93. Brown WJ, Dobson AJ, Mishra G. What is a healthy weight for middle aged women? *Int J Obes Relat Metab Disord* 1998;22:520–8

94. Stevens J. Impact of age on associations between weight and mortality. *Nutr Rev* 2000;58:129–37

95. Lissner L, Bjorkelund C, Heitmann BL, Seidell JC, Bengtsson C. Larger hip circumference independently predicts health and longevity in a Swedish female cohort. *Obes Res* 2001;9:644–6

96. Seidell JC, Perusse L, Despres JP, Bouchard C. Waist and hip circumferences have independent and opposite effects on cardiovascular disease risk factors: the Quebec Family Study. *Am J Clin Nutr* 2001;74:315–21

97. Salamone LM, Cauley JA, Black DM, *et al.* Effect of a lifestyle intervention on bone mineral density in premenopausal women: a randomized trial. *Am J Clin Nutr* 1999;70: 97–103

98. Stevens J, Plankey MW, Williamson DF, *et al.* The body mass index–mortality relationship in white and African American women. *Obes Res* 1998;6:268–77

99. Park YW, Allison DB, Heymsfield SB, Gallagher D. Larger amounts of visceral adipose tissue in Asian Americans. *Obes Res* 2001;9:381–7

100. Kamath SK, Hussain EA, Amin D, *et al.* Cardiovascular disease risk factors in 2 distinct ethnic groups: Indian and Pakistani compared with American premenopausal women. *Am J Clin Nutr* 1999;69:621–31

101. Gallagher D, Heymsfield SB, Heo M, Jebb SA, Murgatroyd PR, Sakamoto Y. Healthy percentage body fat ranges: an approach for developing guidelines based on body mass index. *Am J Clin Nutr* 2000;72:694–701

102. Deurenberg P. Universal cut-off BMI points for obesity are not appropriate. *Br J Nutr* 2001;85:135–6

103. Foster GD, Wadden TA, Vogt RA, Brewer G. What is a reasonable weight loss? Patients' expectations and evaluations of obesity treatment outcomes. *J Consult Clin Psychol* 1997; 65:79–85

104. Blackburn G. Effect of degree of weight loss on health benefits. *Obes Res* 1995;3(Suppl 2): 211S–16S

105. Institute of Medicine. *Weighing the Options.* Washington, DC: National Academy Press, 1995

106. National Institutes of Health. *The Practical Guide. Identification, Evaluation, and Treatment of Overweight and Obesity in Adults.* Washington, DC: National Heart, Lung, and Blood Institute, North American Association for the Study of Obesity, 2000:1–77

107. Willett WC, Stampfer MJ. Clinical practice. What vitamins should I be taking, doctor? *N Engl J Med* 2001;345:1819–24

108. Ditschuneit HH, Flechtner-Mors M, Johnson TD, Adler G. Metabolic and weight-loss effects of a long-term dietary intervention in obese patients. *Am J Clin Nutr* 1999;69:198–204

109. Leibel RL, Hirsch J, Appel BE, Checani GC. Energy intake required to maintain body weight is not affected by wide variation in diet composition. *Am J Clin Nutr* 1992;55:350–5

110. Freedman MR, King J, Kennedy E. Popular diets: a scientific review. *Obes Res* 2001;9 (Suppl 1):1S–40S

111. Parks EJ, Hellerstein MK. Carbohydrate-induced hypertriacylglycerolemia: historical perspective and review of biological mechanisms. *Am J Clin Nutr* 2000;71:412–33

112. Baum CL, Brown M. Low-fat, high-carbohydrate diets and atherogenic risk. *Nutr Rev* 2000;58:148–51

113. Clemens LH, Slawson DL, Klesges RC. The effect of eating out on quality of diet in pre-menopausal women. *J Am Diet Assoc* 1999;99: 442–4

114. Glassberg H, Balady GJ. Exercise and heart disease in women: why, how, and how much? *Cardiol Rev* 1999;7:301–8

115. Kohl HW 3rd. Physical activity and cardiovascular disease: evidence for a dose response. *Med Sci Sports Exerc* 2001;33:S472–83; discussion S493–4

116. Will JC, Massoudi B, Mokdad A, *et al.* Reducing risk for cardiovascular disease in uninsured women: combined results from two WISEWOMAN projects. *J Am Med Womens Assoc* 2001;56:161–5

117. Lichtenstein AH, Kennedy E, Barrier P, *et al.* Dietary fat consumption and health. *Nutr Rev* 1998;56:S3–19; discussion S19–28

118. James WP. A public health approach to the problem of obesity. *Int J Obes Relat Metab Disord* 1995;19(Suppl 3):S37–45

119. Martinez JA. Body-weight regulation: causes of obesity. *Proc Nutr Soc* 2000;59:337–45

120. Zurlo F, Ferraro RT, Fontvielle AM, Rising R, Bogardus C, Ravussin E. Spontaneous physical activity and obesity: cross-sectional and longitudinal studies in Pima Indians. *Am J Physiol* 1992;263:E296–300

121. Wing RR, Hill JO. Successful weight loss maintenance. *Annu Rev Nutr* 2001;21:323–41

122. Schmidt WD, Biwer CJ, Kalscheuer LK. Effects of long versus short bout exercise on fitness and weight loss in overweight females. *J Am Coll Nutr* 2001;20:494–501

123. NIH Consensus Development Panel on Physical Activity and Cardiovascular Health. Physical activity and cardiovascular health. *J Am Med Assoc* 1996;276:241–6

124. Brodney S, McPherson RS, Carpenter RS, Welten D, Blair SN. Nutrient intake of physically fit and unfit men and women. *Med Sci Sports Exerc* 2001;33:459–67

125. Cavagnini F, Croci M, Putignano P, Petroni ML, Invitti C. Glucocorticoids and neuro-endocrine function. *Int J Obes Relat Metab Disord* 2000;24(Suppl 2):S77–9

126. Epel E, Lapidus R, McEwen B, Brownell K. Stress may add bite to appetite in women: a laboratory study of stress-induced cortisol and eating behavior. *Psychoneuroendocrinology* 2001;26:37–49

127. Oliver G, Wardle J, Gibson EL. Stress and food choice: a laboratory study. *Psychosom Med* 2000;62:853–65

128. Wardle J, Steptoe A, Oliver G, Lipsey Z. Stress, dietary restraint and food intake. *J Psychosom Res* 2000;48:195–202

129. Bjorntorp P. Heart and soul: stress and the metabolic syndrome. *Scand Cardiovasc J* 2001; 35:172–7

130. Bjorntorp P, Rosmond R. Obesity and cortisol. *Nutrition* 2000;16:924–36

Hormonal management of symptoms   15

J. L. Chervenak

Approximately 50% of perimenopausal women report acute symptoms including vasomotor instability consisting of hot flashes, night sweats, mood swings and sleep disturbance[1,2]. However, symptoms associated with the perimenopause are often vague, broad and generally non-specific. Irritability and fatigue have been identified as features of the perimenopause but can have many different causes, and are not necessarily due to hormonal fluctuations[3]. The two chief clinical presentations are excessive or frequent bleeding and hot flashes or other symptoms.

As we evaluate the literature, we must be aware of the large difference in the reporting of symptoms between population-based and clinic-based cohorts. A longitudinal analysis of perimenopausal symptoms noted that with time, complaints of headache and breast tenderness decrease while complaints of hot flashes, night sweats and urogenital atrophy increase[4].

Sleep and fatigue

Hot flashes can be disturbing not only during the day but also during sleep. The resulting disturbances in sleep quality may not only lead to subsequent fatigue, but also to changes in mood, memory, irritability, socialization and interpersonal relationships. It is important to remember, however, that we cannot always attribute fatigue to night sweats resulting from hot flashes. Diseases can also have their onset during the perimenopause. The accompanying climacteric changes in mood, sleep and fatigue may act as confounders in the diagnoses of other conditions like hypothyroidism, diabetes, sleep apnea, chronic fatigue syndrome, primary adrenal failure, depression and Cushing's disease.

Hot flashes

Hot flashes are the most common presenting symptom of the climacteric. Every woman, if she lives long enough, will undergo the menopausal transition, either naturally or surgically. While hot flashes are reported all over the world, there are differences in frequencies between countries. The incidence of reported hot flashes associated with spontaneous menopause range from 60% in a Swedish study[5] to 82% in an American study population[6]. Women in developing countries report fewer symptoms than in industrialized countries[7]. It appears that not only hormonal changes but also sociocultural factors play a role in symptoms associated with the maturing woman.

Hot flashes occur with decreases in the estrogenic milieu. Thus the perimenopause, with its 'rollercoaster' estrogen levels, is often accompanied by hot flashes. However, other causative factors may exist, which are still being investigated. Hormonal levels may not play an exclusive role for all women. Studies looking at plasma urinary and vaginal hormone levels found similar levels in postmenopausal women with and without hot flashes[8,9]. This suggests that for some women, other causative factors may also play a role in triggering symptoms.

Agents such as yohimbine, which increase sympathetic activation, can induce hot flashes. They cause a narrower thermoneutral zone, which is the core body temperature at which neither sweating, peripheral vasodilatation, nor shivering can occur[10]. This might explain why stressful situations may invoke hot flashes in some women.

Other agents, like clonidine, which decrease sympathetic activation widen the thermoneutral zone and increase the core body sweating threshold[11]. This may be the mechanism by which relaxation techniques improve complaints regarding hot flashes.

Research is ongoing to increase understanding of the etiology of hot flashes. For example, if sympathetic activation is established as a causative factor in hot flashes, then drugs, which decrease sympathetic activation, like clonidine, but are not associated with hypotension, sedation or other not well-tolerated side-effects, may be useful in the future.

Hormonal therapy and hot flashes

Estrogen therapy is an effective therapy for hot flashes for many women, although the mechanism is still unclear. Freedman and Black noted that estradiol raised the core body temperature sweating threshold and reduced hot flash occurrence in symptomatic postmenopausal woman without changing basal core body temperature or mean skin temperature[12]. If hot flashes do not respond to hormonal therapy, then other conditions such as panic disorders, hyperventilation, diabetic autonomic dysfunction or even carcinoid syndrome or pheochromocytoma might be considered in the differential diagnosis.

Hormonal treatment of vasomotor symptoms includes oral contraceptive pills and hormone replacement therapy (HRT). Relief of vasomotor symptoms should be achieved within 2–3 months of commencing hormonal therapy.

During the perimenopause, some ovarian activity still exists, although the number of functional eggs present is greatly reduced. This is in contrast to the postmenopausal years, when there are no longer any functional eggs. Thus, during the perimenopause, there is a still intact hypothalamic–pituitary–ovarian axis with a diminished number of functional eggs. As a result, follicle stimulating hormone (FSH) and estradiol levels fluctuate

and a veritable estrogen 'rollercoaster' exists. If a woman is at a low point in estrogen, or hypoestrogenic, then hormone replacement doses of estrogen (with or without a progestin depending on presence or absence of a uterus) may ameliorate her resultant vasomotor symptoms. However, if she is at a time period when she is hyperestrogenic, then adding hormone replacement dose therapy may not turn off the hypothalamic–pituitary–ovarian axis and instead may make a subsequent fall in estrogen more precipitous and therefore worsen vasomotor symptoms, bleeding, etc.

Progestins and hot flashes

Depomedroxyprogesterone (DMPA) has been shown to attain a reduction in hot flashes similar to that obtained with estrogen[13,14]. Another progestin, megestrol acetate (Megace®) has been studied in randomized, placebo-controlled studies. Daily doses of 40 mg megestrol have been associated with an 85% reduction in hot flashes[15]. The decrease in hot flashes persisted over time even when the dose was decreased. A possible intolerance issue is the associated increase in appetite sometimes seen with megestrol. Megestrol is also given to cancer patients as an appetite stimulant. A comparative 6-week study of 500 mg DMPA on days 1, 14 and 28 compared with daily 40 mg oral megestrol in 71 women with breast cancer, noted an 89% decrease in hot flash frequency and severity in both groups. These women on DMPA experienced relief from hot flashes for up to 6 months from the time of randomization[16].

Questions exist regarding the long-term effects of DMPA on bone. One year of DMPA use was associated with a significant decrease in lumbar spine bone mineral density (BMD), measured by dual-energy X-ray absorptiometry (DEXA), compared with oral contraceptives or non-hormonal contraception, in a randomized, placebo-controlled study of 155 women aged 18–33 years. After 1 year, DMPA had a significant loss of 2.74%, compared with women not using hormonal contraceptives[17].

Longer-term, cross-sectional studies have shown that prior use of DMPA did not have a measurable impact on BMD[18,19]. Therefore, short-term BMD changes may not translate into long-term clinical significance. However, a large, multicenter, long-term prospective study evaluating BMD after DMPA use should provide more definite conclusions.

Other concerns exist regarding the role of progestins in breast cancer. The Women's Health Initiative (WHI) and other studies have associated the use of medroxyprogesterone acetate with an increased breast cancer risk[20–22]. The use of progestational agents alone for amelioration of hot flash symptoms is a decision that each woman must make for herself, with the guidance of her health-care provider.

Oral contraceptive pills and hot flashes

For a healthy non-smoker, without contraindication, oral contraceptives (combined estrogen with progestin) are underutilized and highly efficacious for relief of vasomotor symptoms. Randomized data support the use of a 20 μg ethinylestradiol/1 mg norethindrone acetate oral contraceptive pill not only for contraception, but also for cycle regulation, relief of vasomotor symptoms and improved quality of life[23]. The higher doses of estrogen in an oral contraceptive, compared to the amount of estrogen in standard HRT, are sufficient to suppress the hypothalamic–pituitary–ovarian axis and therefore prevent the fluctuating estrogen levels seen with the perimenopausal estrogen rollercoaster, and therefore ameliorate hot flashes.

During the perimenopause, oral contraceptives may have other benefits, such as bone benefits, especially in hypoestrogenic women, and prevention of endometrial and ovarian cancer.

Bone loss may accelerate prior to menopause, but this is still an area of research[24]. Oral contraceptives, especially those with more androgenic progestins, may have bone benefits. A Swedish case–control study showed reduction in hip fracture in women who used oral contraception with androgenic progestins after age 40[25]. Another study had similar results regarding possible beneficial bone effects regarding oral contraceptives with androgen-derived progestins. This randomized, placebo-controlled study of women 18–33 years of age, demonstrated that women on norethindrone-containing oral contraceptives had a 2.33% increase in lumbar spine DEXA. Those on a desogestrel-containing oral contraceptive had an increase of 0.33%. The increase in BMD seen on DEXA was significant only for the norethindrone-containing oral contraceptive and not for the less androgenic desogestrel oral contraceptive[17]. How this increase in bone density relates to fracture risk remains unanswered. The greatest effect on BMD may occur when oral contraceptives are used by hypoestrogenic, including at times, perimenopausal women.

Maturing women are at increased risk for gynecological malignancies such as endometrial and ovarian cancer. Compelling evidence exists that oral contraceptives decrease these malignancy rates by 50% and 70%, respectively[26,27]. Oral contraceptives are progestin dominant and therefore protect the endometrium from estrogen's potential effects.

Low-dose oral contraceptive formulations appear to provide similar benefits regarding protection against ovarian cancer to higher-dose oral contraceptives[28]. The mechanism of the protective effect of oral contraceptives regarding ovarian cancer may not be by prevention of incessant ovulation, but, instead, may be due to the effect of the progestin component on ovarian epithelial cell apoptosis[29]. However, the mechanism of oral contraceptives' protective role remains to be elucidated. The role of progestins is an area of great interest, especially since recent publications suggest that estrogen replacement alone may be associated with ovarian cancer incidence[30,31].

Two recent studies provide additional support that there is a link between oral contraceptive use and prevention of ovarian cancer, especially with higher-potency progestins[32]. Also, women with a familial history of ovarian cancer who have used oral contraceptives for

4 or more years had a significantly decreased risk of ovarian cancer at age 70[33].

Measuring hormone levels on hormonal therapy

Hormonal therapy medications in postmenopausal women may produce very different hormone levels in different women. Not only does it vary according to type of medication, but also any woman may have different responses. Thus, it is especially difficult, and potentially misleading, during the perimenopause, to measure hormone levels and use these levels to customize patient care. The physiological processes associated with the perimenopause are too dynamic to evaluate therapy based on blood hormone levels, at any one time. Instead, adjusting therapy based on symptomatology may be more reasonable.

When to adjust dose

While patients often want immediate relief of their symptoms, customization of therapy may take more time. While amelioration of hot flashes is often achieved in 6–8 weeks, it may be more prudent to consider 3 months on hormonal therapy before changing dose or type of medication.

Fertility in the perimenopause

While spontaneous conception after age 45 is very rare, at less than 1% per cycle, it is not impossible[34]. Oral contraceptives and intrauterine devices (IUD)/systems (IUS) offer excellent contraceptive efficacy. While DMPA may be an effective form of contraception, some concerns regarding its long-term effects on bone exist, as discussed above. The contraceptive efficacy of HRT has not been established during the perimenopause. While the likelihood of spontaneous conception is greatly diminished, it is still a consideration. Due to fluctuations in FSH and estradiol during this time, the chance exists for spontaneous conception with a multiple gestation pregnancy. While some hormone replacement regimens may at times suppress ovulation, at other times they may not suppress the hypothalamic–pituitary–ovarian axis for consistent contraceptive needs.

Non-hormonal management of hot flashes

For women who cannot or do not want to use hormonal therapy, options include behavior modification, antidepressants and clonidine.

Behavioral modification includes keeping a symptom diary in order to understand what induces and ameliorates hot flashes, for example, layering clothing, keeping cool and avoiding spicy food, alcohol and caffeine. Stress management, paced respirations and relaxation techniques may also be useful when awake, especially when a woman senses an impending hot flash. Relaxation and deep abdominal breathing (6–8 breaths per minute) have been shown to decrease hot flashes by about 40%[35,36].

When evaluating any study regarding relief of hot flashes, it is important to recognize that in placebo-controlled studies, placebo alone is associated with an approximately 20–30% decrease in hot flashes[37].

Antidepressant therapies can also play a role in relief of vasomotor symptoms. Venlafaxine (Efexor®) is a combined serotonin and norepinephrine re-uptake inhibitor, which has been found to decrease the frequency and severity of hot flashes in a 2-week placebo-controlled, randomized trial. Doses of 75 mg/day of venlafaxine decreased hot flashes by an average of 60%[38]. A longer-term, 8-week follow-up study using open-label venlafaxine (75 mg/day) supported these findings. The 60% decrease in hot flashes persisted throughout the longer study period, without an increase in toxicity[39]. Side-effects of the 75-mg dose included dry mouth, loss of appetite and nausea, which improved with time.

In patients with moderate to severe hot flashes that are affecting daily living and for whom hormonal therapy is not an option, a trial of venlafaxine may be warranted. For these patients, venlafaxine 37.5 mg is recommended for the first week (with food). Hot flashes should be ameliorated by the second week of therapy. If vasomotor symptoms persist, then the dose can be adjusted up to 75 mg, depending on response.

Fluoxetine HCl (Prozac®) is a selective serotonin re-uptake inhibitor (SSRI) type of antidepressant. In a 4-week placebo-controlled trial of 81 women with a history of, or at risk for, breast cancer was associated with a 50% decrease in hot flashes, compared with 36% in the placebo arm[40].

Other agents have also been associated in relief of vasomotor symptoms including clonidine and bellergal. Despite its widespread use, especially in past years, clonidine can have intolerable side-effects including hypotension, fatigue, constipation, drowsiness, insomnia and dry mouth. Clonidine was associated with a 45% reduction in hot flashes compared to 25% in the placebo group[37,41].

Bellergal is a combination of phenobarbital and belladonna alkaloids, which was used more frequently in the past. It has potential intolerance problems given its components, including nausea. Today's newer non-hormonal agents relieve symptoms better and are safer.

Dysfunctional uterine bleeding in the perimenopause

Irregular bleeding can be a significant problem during the perimenopause. Not only does it present as a health issue, but it can also affect quality of life. Many surgical procedures, including dilatation and curettage, and hysterectomy are performed during the perimenopausal years when hormonal fluctuations may cause exacerbation of symptoms. Before commencing any type of hormonal therapy for irregular bleeding in the perimenopausal years, other causes of abnormal bleeding should be excluded. During the menopausal transition, hyperestrogenemia, inadequate progesterone production and acyclic secretion of estrogen[42] may predispose a woman to endometrial hyperplasia or carcinoma. Appropriate evaluation might consist of an endometrial biopsy, dilatation and curettage, hysteroscopy or transvaginal ultrasound with saline infusion sonohysterography (SIS).

Transvaginal ultrasound is best performed after spontaneous menses or induced withdrawal bleeding so that only the 1-mm thick basalis layer is present in a normal uterus[43]. SIS can enhance specificity of the thickness of the endometrial image. Virtually all lesions observed on hysteroscopy or hysterectomy were visible by SIS in more than 90 studies[44]. Nonetheless, the capabilities of the sonographer are an important consideration. SIS is usually well tolerated by patients who generally prefer it to office hysteroscopy[45].

Once a mechanical etiology of the bleeding has been ruled out (polyps, submucous myomas, malignancy, etc.), hormonal therapy can be instituted. The two goals of hormonal treatment of dysfunctional uterine bleeding (DUB) are to stabilize the endometrium and to prevent 'rollercoaster' levels of FSH with hyperestrogenism and low progesterone. While progestin-only therapy may be sufficient as a temporal measure to stabilize the endometrium, it is not sufficient for stabilization of FSH. Oral contraceptives, with their higher estrogen dosage than HRT (0.625 mg conjugated equine estrogen has equivalent potency to 5–10 µg ethinylestradiol with regard to bone density[46]), better achieve the two goals for healthy non-smoking perimenopausal women, without contraindication.

Acute therapy of perimenopausal DUB

If the bleeding results from hyperestrogenism, then progestin administration would stabilize the proliferative endometrium. This could be achieved with some type of hormonal therapy, such as a progestin-dominant oral contraceptive pill, oral micronized progesterone 200 mg/day for 10 days or medroxyprogesterone acetate 10 mg/day for 10 days. Once the progestin component is withdrawn or completed, a very heavy menses may occur due to prior endometrial overgrowth from the hyperestrogenic environment.

If a woman complains of menorrhagia, then use of estrogen alone (oral or transdermal) may help achieve endometrial stabilization[47].

Long-term management of perimenopausal DUB

In a perimenopausal female with DUB, resulting from hormonal fluctuations with time periods of elevated FSH, hyperestrogenism and low progesterone, the use of progestin alone, in most tolerated doses, does not provide sufficient negative feedback on FSH to prevent the 'rollercoaster' effects on bleeding. A low-dose estrogen with progestin oral contraceptive, in an appropriate candidate, is an excellent option. Continuous oral contraceptives with withdrawals every 3–6 months offer good cycle control. If a woman's irregular bleeding is improved but persistant on a 20-µg ethinylestradiol contraceptive, and she has a thin atrophic endometrium visualized on transvaginal ultrasound, then she may benefit from increasing the dose of a still low-dose, continuous, monophasic oral contraceptive. Oral contraceptives are progestin dominant and are associated with a decidualized and atrophic endometrium. However, breakthrough bleeding may occur if there is too much endometrial atrophy. The higher dose of the still low-dose oral contraceptive (30–35 µg) might better stabilize her endometrium. Choice of a continuous, monophasic oral contraceptive may minimize symptoms resulting from fluctuations in hormonal levels, including bleeding and hot flashes.

If a woman cannot tolerate, or is not a candidate for, an oral contraceptive, then she may benefit from a combined continuous HRT. She is more likely to achieve success with this type of regimen if she has had at least 6 months of amenorrhea.

Progestin-only therapy for DUB

Cyclic administration of medroxyprogesterone acetate has been shown not to be an effective therapy for perimenopausal irregular bleeding[48].

For patients intolerant of estrogen, a progestin-only oral contraceptive might be considered. However, this may result in lower estradiol levels, which may lead to subsequent future bone loss. Higher doses of progestin may provide some endometrial control with some FSH control as well; however, these doses often have intolerable side-effects.

Progestin IUDs for DUB

Progestin IUDs or IUS (Mirena®) offer not only improvements regarding bleeding but also provide contraception. In a prospective 12-month, randomized study of postmenopausal women on estrogen replacement therapy, IUDs containing 10 or 20 µg/day of levonorgestrel had higher amenorrhea rates than 5 mg/day of sequential medroxyprogesterone acetate. Neither of the IUDs was associated with endometrial hyperplasia. The 10-µg IUD had higher acceptance rates (98.2% vs. 86.2% for the 20-µg IUD and 81.6% for medroxyprogesterone acetate)[49].

Hormonally associated headaches in the perimenopause

Fluctuating levels of circulating estradiol may not only be associated with perimenopausal hot flashes and DUB, but also with migraine headaches, especially if the patient has a history of hormonally associated headaches (i.e. menstrual migraines).

Menstrual migraines occur with falls in circulating estradiol concentrations[50], while luteal phase progesterone levels have no effect[51]. The perimenopause, with its 'rollercoaster' estrogen levels may predispose a woman to hormonally associated headaches.

For a healthy perimenopausal non-smoking woman, with migraine headaches and without contraindication to oral contraceptive hormonal therapy, a low-dose (20 µg ethinylestradiol) oral contraceptive given at bedtime, with a lower lose of estrogen given instead during the placebo week, has been associated with symptom relief[52]. However, she may achieve even better symptom relief with a continuous low-dose oral contraceptive without any decrease in the placebo week.

Bedtime administration of oral contraceptives or oral HRT is important for migraine sufferers. The lowest threshold for migraines occurs in the morning and a major migraine trigger is dropping estradiol levels.

Transdermal estrogen therapy is another option, especially for those patients especially sensitive to hormonal fluctuations or those for whom an oral contraceptive is contraindicated. A transdermal 0.1-mg 17β-estradiol patch has been found to have a similar efficacy to estradiol gel for menstrual migraine prophylaxis[53]. The patch can be applied 2 days before the expected menses or 1 day before the anticipated menses. If headaches occur the day before the patch change on weekly transdermal therapy consider a biweekly patch.

While concerns have existed regarding the use of the higher-estrogen dose oral contraceptives of the past and the incidence of stroke, today's lower-dose oral contraceptives do not seem to have the same association in a healthy, non-smoking normotensive woman[54]. However, if concerns exist regarding the etiology of the headaches, defer any type of hormonal therapy until a diagnosis is made.

Skin changes with aging

During the perimenopause, many changes occur, some of which can be cosmetically distressing, such as the appearance of thinner, drier, wrinkled skin, especially in our youth-oriented society. An Austrian study of 24 women, mean age 54.9 years, studied skin changes after 6 months of treatment with either transdermal estrogen, transdermal or oral estrogen with a vaginal progestin, or an unblinded control group receiving no therapy. They observed that women in any of the hormonal therapy arms had significant improvements in skin lipids, skin elasticity, skin thickness and skin surface lipids compared with the control group[55]. The end result of a thicker dermis and less dry skin may be desirable by some women.

Depression in the perimenopause

Depression is not more common during the menopause transition[56]. However, if a woman has a history of depression, she may be sensitive to associated symptoms such as mood changes[57] and fatigue. Although separate entities, these two conditions can co-exist and may act as confounders to each other when establishing a correct diagnosis. Therefore, presence or absence of an undiagnosed depressive disorder must always be determined. If depression exists, then it must be treated independently from issues related to perimenopausal cycle control.

Depression with premenstrual syndrome in the perimenopause

We do not yet understand the causative factors of perimenopausal premenstrual syndrome (PMS). However, high luteal phase estrogen has been associated with increased PMS symptoms[58]. During perimenopause, there are periods of hyperestrogenism. This may predispose susceptible women to PMS symptoms.

While it is commonly believed that progestins depress mood, a placebo-controlled study of non-depressed, early postmenopausal women showed no difference in mood after 2 weeks of conjugated equine estrogen, conjugated equine estrogen with 5 mg medroxyprogesterone acetate, or conjugated equine estrogens with 200 mg micronized progesterone[59]. The study may not have been long enough, however, for the progestins to have mood effects. There was more reported breast tenderness and vaginal bleeding in the medroxyprogesterone users than in the micronized progesterone users. These factors may act as confounders concerning mood, libido, etc.

Thyroid screening in the perimenopause

Thyroid disease may present with many of the same symptoms of perimenopause, such as difficulties with sleep, mood, fatigue and irritability. Therefore, thyroid disease should be included in the differential diagnosis. Although there is no agreement on whether universal thyroid stimulating hormone (TSH) screening should be carried out, the perimenopause presents an ideal opportunity. A cost-effectiveness analysis concluded that after age 35, independent of symptoms, thyroid screening should be done once every 5 years[60].

Sexual well-being in the perimenopause

During the menopause transition, women face significant emotional and physical changes which may impact on their sexual health. For some, irregular bleeding, fatigue, hot flashes, dyspareunia, irritability and other perimenopausal symptoms may affect libido. A common cause for sexual dissatisfaction in the maturing women is lack of a partner, from divorce or death. It is important that the health-care provider address these and other factors, which may be associated with their sexual health.

Patients often want a pill that will act as a panacea for all their problems, including decreased libido. The media have given much press to the benefits of androgens, and yet hormones may not be the causative factors for changes in libido, in some patients. Instead, for some, night sweats and disturbed sleep may affect a woman's sense of well-being and may deprive her of her perceived sexual drive. These factors must be evaluated before any type of hormonal therapy is begun. A symptom diary may help pinpoint causes for decreased libido for some patients. For example, one patient presented requesting androgens for her decreased libido. On intake history, initially, she vehemently denied that her decreased libido was associated with her spousal relationship. After keeping her diary, she was able to make an association between arguments regarding television and in-laws and successfully adjust her behavior so that she was able to improve her libido without any type of androgen therapy.

However, for some women, testosterone levels can change during perimenopause, menopause or postmenopause[61]. For patients with low free testosterone levels and severe menopausal symptoms, especially low libido

and energy, whose symptoms are not relieved with estrogen or estrogen with progestin, then androgen therapy might be considered. Androgens are most useful for women who have had oophorectomy prior to natural menopause. However, more research is needed regarding the safety of long-term androgen use.

Potential problems associated with androgens include its negative effect on serum lipids, hirsutism, aggressive behavior and permanent voice deepening. Although androgens can be given alone, doses can be lowered when combined with estrogen and, therefore, negative effects may be reduced.

Alternative therapies

Alternative medicine has been defined as '...medical interventions that are neither widely taught in US medical school nor generally available in US hospitals'[62]. However, these 'natural' therapies are what many of our patients are using for amelioration of perimenopausal symptoms. The highest rates of use of these therapies during the perimenopausal and early postmenopausal years[63] are 42% and 44% for ages 35–49 and 50–64 years, respectively.

Common alternative therapies for relief of perimenopausal symptoms include black cohosh, dong quai, soy, chasteberry, red clover, Siberian ginseng, vitamin E, evening primrose oil, St. John's wort and wild yam cream.

Women often turn to 'natural or alternative' therapies because they think that they are a safe way to ameliorate symptoms. However, if they are effective in relieving symptoms, then they may have hormonal activity. In 1994, the Dietary Supplement Health and Education Act was instituted. Manufacturers were responsible for the safety of their products. However, supplements were defined as neither food nor drug and were not identified as needing Food and Drug Administration (FDA) approval. However, their supposed safety is assumed, and not proven.

One of women's greatest fears is of getting breast cancer. A total of 38% of women perceive that breast cancer will be their cause of death, while their actual lifetime risk may be 4%[64]. In *in vivo* studies of the human breast cancer cell line MCF-7, and in oophorectomized mice, dong quai and ginseng induced the growth of MCF-7 cells by 16- and 27-fold, respectively, over that of untreated control cells. These same herbs did not show activation of human estrogen receptor α or human estrogen receptor β, and did not affect *in vivo* mouse uterine weight after 4 days. This suggests that dong quai and ginseng may stimulate growth of the human breast cancer cell line MCF-7, independent of estrogenic activity. Therefore, women should be cautious about using these therapies during or to prevent breast cancer until further study[65].

Black cohosh

Black cohosh (*Cimicifuga racemosa*), known in tablet form as Remifemin, is a herb from the root of a plant used by native North American Indians[63]. It has been used for centuries in the treatment of women's reproductive disorders and is among the most widely used of alternative therapies for the management of vasomotor symptoms. It is widely prescribed in Germany where it is used as a treatment for depression, sleep disturbances and hot flashes. In Germany it is regulated, unlike in the USA.

Some placebo-controlled trials demonstrate that black cohosh and soy may ameliorate symptoms for some women. However, for most women, they do not appear to be as effective as hormonal therapy. Black cohosh does not appear to affect bone. Randomized, placebo-controlled studies regarding long-term efficacy, safety and side-effects have not yet been published[66]. The mechanism of action for the purported relief of vasomotor symptoms has yet to be elucidated and its actual efficacy is in question. Many non-placebo-controlled studies outside the USA are published in the German Commission E Monographs and suggest that black cohosh is effective in management of hot flashes. However, a placebo-controlled, randomized US trial ($n = 85$), of breast cancer patients on

tamoxifen, found that black cohosh was no more effective than placebo in reducing hot flashes, although it did reduce sweating[67].

Dong quai

In randomized clinical trial data, dong quai was no more helpful than placebo in relieving menopausal symptoms[68]. However, this is a common over-the-counter preparation, which is often used in combination with other therapies. It has coumarin-like activity and caution should be taken for those patients on anticoagulant therapy.

Chasteberry

The proposed mechanism of action of chasteberry in the German Commission E Monographs is by binding to androgen receptors and creating an antiandrogenic environment. It also inhibits prolactin and prevents progesterone insufficiency. While the decrease in prolactin may potentially help regarding breast tenderness, the mechanism by which chasteberry relieves other perimenopausal symptoms is unclear.

St. John's wort

St. John's wort is commonly used for mild/moderate depression, anxiety, seasonal affective disorders and sleep disorders. In Germany it is prescribed 20 times more often than Prozac. It does not appear to be effective, however, in the treatment of major depressive disorder. A double-blind, randomized, placebo multicenter trial of the effect of St. John's wort in major depressive disorder failed to demonstrate the efficacy in relieving symptoms better than placebo[69]. However, it is for mild depressive symptoms that women often self-medicate.

While it is standardized to its hypericin component, its mechanism of action remains unclear. It is postulated to have a monoamine oxidase (MAO)-like effect and/or to interact with serotonin.

In March 2000, the UK Department of Health issued a warning about St. John's wort:

'The Medicines which may be affected by St. John's Wort include some medications for the treatment of HIV (AZT) … heart conditions (digitalis and digoxin) … asthma (theophyline) and the oral contraceptive pill.'

Vitamin E

Observational studies suggest that vitamin E may be beneficial for cardiac disease prevention and cancer outcomes. It is essentially safe, unless excessive quantities are consumed and relatively inexpensive. However, regarding hot flashes, a randomized clinical trial showed vitamin E to be ineffective for relief of vasomotor symptoms[70].

Red clover

Extracts of red clover (*Trifolium pratense*) are one of the commonly used herbal therapies promoted for relief of vasomotor symptoms as a source for phytoestrogens, and therefore a 'natural' form of HRT. It is in the top 5% of 150 herbs tested in a binding assay for progesterone and estradiol[71]. In animal studies, red clover produces estrogenic effects including enlargement of the vulva, uterus, udder and teats[72]. In Australia in the 1940s, there was an epidemic of 'clover disease' when grazing sheep consuming *Trifolium subterraneum* were noted to experience infertility and abnormal lactation. Like red clover, subterranean clover contains large amounts of phytoestrogens[73].

Two double-blind, placebo-controlled studies were designed to evaluate whether or not red clover was beneficial for relieving menopausal symptoms. Neither found red clover extract to be of benefit[74,75]. Three trials[76–78] showed no significant increase in endometrial thickness after less than 6 months of exposure to red clover. It has been suggested that isoflavones may have an antiproliferative effect on the endometrium compared to estrogen. However, a randomized, placebo-controlled clinical study of red clover using immunohistochemical proliferation markers did not demonstrate an antiproliferative effect on the endometrium[79]. Therefore, the question regarding long-term safety of red clover persists. Longer study periods are necessary to determine effects on endometrial stimulation[80].

Another potential concern regarding red clover is that some clover species have coumarins, and microorganisms can act on the clover to produce dicoumarol, an anticoagulant from which warfarin anticoagulants were derived[80,81]. No published studies to date have investigated the potential role of coumarins on tests of blood clotting and coagulation.

Soy

Observational studies suggest that soy-based diets have numerous benefits including an improved lipoprotein profile compared to an animal protein diet, decrease in fracture risk and relief of menopausal symptoms[82–84].

While epidemiological studies suggest that Japanese women living in Japan have a decreased number of reproductive cancers, this benefit is lost when they migrate to Hawaii and further lost when they migrate to the mainland USA. A causative factor may be the type of soy used in Japan compared with that in the US mainland. In Japan, women tend to eat more fermented soy products in a lower-fat, lower-calorie diet rich in omega 3 fatty acids. They also consume significantly more daily isoflavones than are consumed in the USA. However, soy is more than just isoflavones, it also consists of coumestans and lignans. Alcohol processing of soy's isoflavones removes biologically active forms. The soy milk, tofu products and homogenized isoflavone tablets commonly purchased in the supermarket and health food store may not necessarily have the same actions as those consumed by Japanese women living in Japan.

While some studies suggest benefits from soy regarding relief from hot flashes, other studies have conflicting results. A placebo-controlled, randomized, double-blind study ($n = 80$) of women (average age 49 years) showed that 4 months of divided-dose therapy of 100 mg/day of isoflavones, was associated with significant improvements in perimenopausal symptoms (hot flashes, weakness, insomnia and headache)[85]. A randomized, placebo-controlled study ($n = 155$) used a dose equivalent to 150 mg of soy isoflavones once a day for 4 weeks. No difference was found compared to placebo[86]. Another randomized, placebo-controlled study ($n = 177$) also used a dose equivalent to 150 mg of soy isoflavones for 12 weeks. While hot flash frequency was noted to be decreased compared with placebo at 6 weeks, there was no difference at 12 weeks[87]. The current consensus of the North American Menopause Society is that data concerning soy and hot flashes are inconclusive[88].

Wild yam cream

Proponents of wild yam cream claim it is a 'natural source of DHEA [dehydroepiandrosterone] and progesterone'. These topical creams are commonly sold in health food stores and over the Internet as an alternative to progesterone. Claims are made that it can increase libido, improve bone density, prevent breast and endometrial cancer, and substitute for prescribed hormonal therapy.

However, there is no human biochemical conversion pathway from the diosgenin in wild yam to a usable form of progesterone in the body. To date, no prospective, randomized, double-blinded studies exist which have the power to overcome the confounders in the studies. No appropriate clinical trials have been performed to determine whether the over-the-counter progesterone creams even contain enough progestin to alter hormone blood levels or prevent the uterus from overstimulation by estrogen. No valid claims can be made as yet regarding reduction in rates of endometrial or breast cancer.

References

1. McKinlay SM, Jefferys M. The menopausal syndrome. *Br J Prev Soc Med* 1974;28:109–15
2. Brambilla DJ, McKinlay SM, Johannes CB, *et al*. Defining the perimenopause for application in epidemiologic investigations. *Am J Epidemiol* 1994;140:1091–5
3. The SWAN Research Group Study of Women's Health Across the Nation (SWAN). Menopausal symptoms in an ethnically diverse population of midlife women. *Presented at the 125th Annual Meeting of the American Public Health Association*, Indianapolis, IN November, 1997:abstr 3244
4. Dennerstein L, Dudley EC, Hopper JL, *et al*. A prospective population based study of menopausal symptoms. *Obstet Gynecol* 1998;19:165–73
5. Hagstad A, Janson PO. The epidemiology of climacteric symptoms. *Acta Obstet Gynecol Scand* 1986;134(Suppl):59–65
6. Feldman BM, Voda A, Gronseth E, *et al*. The prevalence of hot flashes and associated variables among postmenopausal women. *Res Nurs Health* 1985;8:261–8
7. Obermeyer CM. Menopause across cultures: a review of the evidence. *Menopause* 2000;7:184–92
8. Askel S, Schomberg DW, Tyrey L, *et al*. Vasomotor symptoms, serum estrogens and gonadotropin levels in surgical menopause. *Am J Obstet Gynecol* 1976;126:165–9
9. Stone SC, Mickal A, Rye F, *et al*. Postmenopausal symptomatology maturation index and plasma estrogen levels. *Obstet Gynecol* 1975;45:625–7
10. Freedman RR, Woodward S, Sabharwal SC. Alpha 2-adrenergic mechanism in menopausal hot flushes. *Obstet Gynecol* 1990;76:573–9
11. Freedman RR, Dinsay R. Clonidine raises the sweating threshold in symptomatic but not in asymptomatic postmenopausal women. *Fertil Steril* 2000;74:20–3
12. Freedman R, Black C. Estrogen raises the sweating threshold in postmenopausal women with hot flashes. *Fertil Steril* 2002;3:487–90
13. Lobo R, McCormick W, Singer F. DMPA compared with conjugated estrogens for the treatment of postmenopausal women. *Obstet Gynecol* 1984;63:1–5
14. Morrison J, Martin D, Blair R, *et al*. The use of MPA for relief of climacteric symptoms. *Am J Obstet Gynecol* 1980;138:99–104
15. Loprinzi C, Michalak J, Quella S, *et al*. Megestrol acetate for the prevention of hot flashes. *N Engl J Med* 1994;331:347–52
16. Quella S, Loprinzi C, Sloan J, *et al*. Long term use of megestrol acetate by cancer survivors for the treatment of hot flashes. *Cancer* 1998;82:1784–8

17. Berenson A, Radecki C, Grady J, et al. A prospective controlled study of the effects of hormonal contraception on bone mineral density. Obstet Gynecol 2001;98:576–81
18. Petitti DB, Sidney S, Bernstein A, et al. Obstet Gynecol 2000;95:736–44
19. Orr-Walker BJ, Evans MC, Ames RW, et al. The effect of past use of the injectable contraceptive depot medroxyprogesterone acetate on bone mineral density in normal post-menopausal women. Clin Endocrinol 1998;49: 615–18
20. Writing group for the Women's Health Initiative Investigators. Risks and benefits of estrogen plus progestin in healthy post-menopausal women: principal results from the WHI randomized controlled trial. J Am Med Assoc 2002;288:321–33
21. Chen CL, Weiss NS, Newcomb P, et al. HRT in relation to breast cancer. J Am Med Assoc 2002;288:321–33
22. Schairer C, Lubin J, Troisi R, et al. Menopausal estrogen and estrogen–progestin replacement therapy and breast cancer risk. J Am Med Assoc 2000;283:485–91
23. Casper RF, Dodin S, Reid RT, et al. The effect of a 20 µg ethinyl estradiol/1 mg norethindrone acetate low dose oral contraceptive on vaginal bleeding patterns, hot flashes and quality of life in symptomatic perimenopausal women. Menopause 1997;4:139–47
24. Slemenda C, Longcope C, Peakcock M, et al. Sex steroids, bone mass and bone loss in a prospective study of pre-, peri- and post-menopausal women. J Clin Invest 1996;97: 14–21
25. Michaelsson K, Baron JA, Farahmand BY, et al. OC use and risk of hip fracture: a case control study. Lancet 1999;353:1481–4
26. The Cancer and Steroid Hormone Study of the CDC (CASH) and the National Institute of Child Health and Human Development. The reduction in risk of ovarian cancer associated with oral contraceptive use. N Engl J Med 1987;316:650–5
27. The Cancer and Steroid Hormone Study of the CDC (CASH) and the National Institute of Child Health and Human Development. Combination oral contraceptive use and the risk of endometrial cancer. J Am Med Assoc 1987;257:796–800
28 Gnagy S, Ming EE, Devesa SS, et al. Declining ovarian cancer rates in US women in relation to parity and oral contraceptive use. Epidemiology 2000;11:102–5
29. Rodriguez GC, Walmer DH, Cline M, et al. Effect of progestin on the ovarian epithelium of macaques: cancer prevention through apoptosis. J Soc Gynecol Invest 1998;5:271–6
30. Lacey JV, Mink PJ, Lubin JH, et al. Menopausal hormone replacement therapy and risk of ovarian cancer. J Am Med Assoc 2002;288:334–41
31. Rodriguez GC, Patel AV, Calle EE, et al. Hormone replacement therapy and ovarian cancer risk: American Cancer Society Study. J Am Med Assoc 2001;21:1460–5
32. Schildkraut JM, Calingaert B, Marchbanks P, et al. Impact of progestin and estrogen potency in oral contraceptives on ovarian cancer risk. J Natl Cancer Inst 2002;94:32–8
33. Walker GR, Schlesselman JJ, Ness RB. Family history of cancer, oral contraceptive use and ovarian cancer risk. Am J Obstet Gynecol 2002; 186:8–14
34. Menken J. Age at menopause and fecundity preceding menopause. In Gray R, Lendon H, Airia A, eds. Biomedical Determinants of Reproduction. Oxford, UK: Clarendon Press, 1993:65–84
35. Irvin JH, Domar AD, Clark C, et al. The effects of relaxation response training on menopausal symptoms. J Psychosom Obstet Gynecol 1996;17: 202–7
36. Freedman RR, Woodward S. Behavioral treatment of menopausal hot flushes: evaluation by ambulatory monitoring. Am J Obstet Gynecol 1992;167:436–9
37. Sloan JA, Loprinzi CL, Novotny PJ, et al. Methodological lessons learned from hot flash studies. J Clin Oncol 2001;19:4280–90
38. Loprinzi CL, Kugler JW, Sloan JA, et al. Venlafaxine in management of hot flashes in survivors of breast cancer: a randomized controlled trial. Lancet 2000;356:2959–63
39. Barton D, LaVasseur B, Loprinzi C, et al. The use of venlafaxine for hot flashes: results of a longitudinal continuation phase. Oncol Nurs Forum 2002;29:33–40
40. Loprinzi CL, Sloan JA, Perez EA, et al. Phase 3 evaluation of fluoxetine for treatment of hot flashes. J Clin Oncol 2002;20:1578–83
41. Pandya KJ, Raubertas R, Flynn P, et al. Oral clonidine in postmenopausal patients with breast cancer experiencing tamoxifen induced hot flashes. J Clin Oncol 1994;12:155–8
42. Santoro N, Brown JR, Adel T, et al. Characterization of reproductive hormonal dynamics in the perimenopause. J Clin Endocrinol Metab 1996;81:1495–1501
43. Goldstein SR, Zeltser I, Horan CK, et al. Ultrasonography based triage for perimenopausal patients with abnormal uterine bleeding. Am J Obstet Gynecol 1997;177:102–8
44. Dijkhuizen FP, DeVries LD, Mol BW, et al. Comparison of transvaginal ultrasonography and SIS for the detection of intracavitary abnormalities in premenopausal women. Ultrasound Obstet Gynecol 2000;15:372–6

45. Timmerman D, Deprest J, Bourne T, *et al.* A randomized trial on the use of ultrasonography of office hysterography for endometrial assessment in postmenopausal patients with breast cancer, treated with tamoxifen. *Am J Obstet Gynecol* 1998;179:62–70

46. Speroff L, Glass R, Kase N. Menopause and postmenopausal hormone therapy. In Speroff L, Glass R, Kase N, eds. *Clinical Gynecologic Endocrinology and Infertility*. Baltimore, MD: Williams and Wilkins, 1994:618–19

47. DeVore GR, Owens O, Kase N, *et al.* Use of IV premarin in the treatment of DUB. *Obstet Gynecol* 1982;59:285–91

48. Letharby A, Irving G, Cameron I, *et al.* Cyclical progestogens for heavy menstrual bleeding. *Cochrane Database Syst Rev* 2000:CD00106

49. Raudaskosk T, Tapanainen J, Tomas E, *et al.* Intrauterine 10 μg and 20 μg levonorgestrel systems in postmenopausal women receiving oral oestrogen replacement therapy: clinical, endometrial and metabolic response. *Br J Obstet Gynaecol* 2002;109:136–44

50. Somerville BW. The role of estradiol withdrawal in the etiology of menstrual migraine. *Neurology* 1972;22:355–65

51. Somerville BW. The role of progestin in menstrual migraine. *Neurology* 1971;21:853

52. Calhoun A. Adjusting estradiol concentration reduces headache frequency and severity in female migraineurs. Presented at the *International Headache Congress*, New York, July 2001

53. Predalier A, Vincent D, Beaulieu PH, *et al.* Correlation between oestradiol plasma level and therapeutic effect on menstrual migraine. In Rose FC, ed. *New Advances in Headache Research*, 4th edn. London: Smith Gordon, 1994:129–32

54. Petitti DB, Signey S, Bernstein A. Stroke in users of low dose oral contraceptives. *N Engl J Med* 1996;335:8–15

55. Sator PG, Schmidt JP, Sator MD, *et al.* The influence of HRT on skin aging: a pilot study. *Maturitas* 2001;39:43–55

56. McKinlay SM, Brambilla DJ, Posner JC, *et al.* The normal menopause transition. *Am J Hum Biol* 1992;4:37–46

57. Harlow BI, Signorello LB. Factors associated with early menopause. *Maturitas* 2000; 35:3–9

58. Seippel L, Backstrom T. Luteal phase estradiol relates to symptom severity in patients with premenstrual syndrome. *J Clin Endocrinol Metab* 1998;83:1988–92

59. Cummings JA, Brizendine L. Comparison of physical and emotional side effects of progesterone or medroxyprogesterone in early postmenopausal women. *Menopause* 2002;9: 253–63

60. Danese MD, Powe NR, Sawin CT, *et al.* Screening for mild thyroid failure at the periodic health examination: a decision and cost-effectiveness analysis. *J Am Med Assoc* 1996;271:285–92

61. Davis S, Burger H. Androgens and the postmenopausal woman. *J Clin Endocrinol Metab* 1996;81:2759–63

62. Eisenberg DM, Davis RB, Ettner SL, *et al.* Trends in alternative medicine use in the United States, 1990–1997: results of a follow-up national survey. *J Am Med Assoc* 1998;280:1569–75

63. Tyler V. *The Honest Herbal*. New York: Pharmaceutical Products Press, 1993

64. Mosca L, Jones WK, King KB, *et al.* Awareness, perception, and knowledge of heart disease risk and prevention among women in the United States. *Arch Fam Med* 2000;9:506–15

65. Amato P, Christophe S, Mellon P, *et al.* Estrogenic activity of herbs commonly used as remedies for menopausal symptoms. *Menopause* 2002;2:145–50

66. Foster S. Black cohosh (*Cimifuga racemosa*): a literature review. *Herbalgram* 1999;45:35–49

67. Jacobson JS, Troxel AB, Evans J. Randomized trial of black cohosh for the treatment of hot flashes among women with a history of breast cancer. *J Clin Oncol* 2001;19:2739–45

68. Hirata JD, Swiersz LM, Zell B, *et al.* Does dong quai have estrogenic effects in postmenopausal women? A double-blind, placebo-controlled trial. *Fertil Steril* 1987;68:981–6

69. Hypericum Depression Trial Study Group. Effect of *Hypericum perforatum* (St John's wort) in major depressive disorder. *J Am Med Assoc* 2002;287:1807–14

70. Barton DL, Loprinzi CL, Ouella SK, *et al.* Prospective evaluation of vitamin E for hot flashes in breast cancer survivors. *J Clin Oncol* 1998;16:495–500

71. Zava DT, Dollbaum CM, Blen M, *et al.* Estrogen and progestin bioactivity of foods, herbs and spices. *Proc Soc Exp Biol Med* 1998;217:369–78

72. Nwannenna AI, Lundh TJ, Omadej A. Clinical changes in ovarectomized ewes exposed to phytoestrogens and 17β estradiol implants. *Proc Soc Exp Biol Med* 1995;208:92–7

73. Lewis RA. *Lewis Dictionary of Toxicology*. Boca Raton, FL: CRC Press, 1998:1067

74. Babar RJ, Templeman C, Morton T. Randomized placebo controlled trial of an isoflavone supplement and menopausal symptoms in women. *Climacteric* 1999;2:85–92

75. Knight DC, Howes JB, Eden JA. The effect of Promensil, an isoflavone extract, on menopausal symptoms. *Climacteric* 1999;2:79–84

76. Babar RJ, Templeman C, Morton T. Randomized placebo controlled trial of an isoflavone

supplement and menopausal symptoms in women. *Climacteric* 1999;2:85–92

77. Nachtigall LE, Nachtigall LB. The effects of isoflavone derived from red clover on vasomotor symptoms and endometrial thickness. In *Proceedings of the 9th International Menopause Society World Congress on the Menopause.* 1999:128 abstr

78. Babar R, Clifton Bligh P, Fulcher G. The effect of an isoflavone extract on serum lipids, forearm bone density and endometrial thickness in postmenopausal women. In *Proceedings of the North American Menopause Society.* 1999:abstr

79. Hale G, Huges C, Robboy S, *et al.* A double-blind randomized study on the effect of red clover isoflavones on the endometrium. *Menopause* 2001;8:338–46

80. Fugh-Berman A, Kronenberg F. Red clover for menopausal women: current state of knowledge. *Menopause* 2001;8:333–7

81. Dewick PM. *Medicinal Natural Products: a Biosynthetic Approach.* West Sussex, UK: John Wiley and Sons, 1997

82. Anderson JW, Johnstone BM, Cook-Newell ME. Meta-analysis of the effects of soy protein intake on serum lipids. *N Engl J Med* 1995; 333:276–82

83. Burke GL. *Curr Opin Endocrinol Diabetes* 1996; 3:508–13

84. Scambia G, Mango D, Signorile PG, *et al.* Clinical effects of standardized soy extract in postmenopausal women: a pilot study. *Menopause* 2000;7:105–11

85. Han KK, Soares JM, Haidar MA, *et al.* Benefits of soy isoflavone therapeutic regimens on menopausal symptoms. *Obstet Gynecol* 2002;99: 389–94

86. Quella SK, Loprinzi CL, Barton DL, *et al.* Evaluation of soy phytoestrogens for treatment of hot flushes in breast cancer survivors. A North Central Cancer treatment group trial. *J Clin Oncol* 2000;10:68–74

87. Upmalis DH, Lobo R, Bradley L, *et al.* Vasomotor symptoms relief by soy isoflavone extract tablets in postmenopausal women: a multicenter, double-blind, randomized placebo-controlled study. *Menopause* 2000;7:236–42

88. North American Menopause Society. Consensus opinion: the role of isoflavones in menopausal health. *Menopause* 2000;7:215–29

Index

abnormal uterine bleeding 69, 149–150
  diagnostic approaches 71–74
  leiomyomas (fibroids) and 69–70, 90–91
  menometrorrhagia 69
  menorrhagia 70, 91, 119
  metrorrhagia 69
  therapy 74–76, 90–91, 99, 149–150
    acute therapy 149
    long-term management 150
    progestin-only therapy 150
abortion, spontaneous 6
activin
  changes during menopause transition 14
  changes with reproductive aging 9
adenomyosis 93–94, 119
affairs 45
age
  at menopause 1, 30
    nutritional effects 127
    significance for health 127
  effect on fertility 6
  testosterone changes 40
aging *see* reproductive aging
alcohol
  abuse 3, 46
  age at menopause and 127
  breast cancer risk and 132
  cardiovascular disease and 130
alternative therapies 152–154
  sexual dysfunction 54–55
amenorrhea 1–2
androgens 39–42
  bioavailability 40–42
  breast cancer risk relationship 51–52
  changes during menopause transition 15, 42
  insufficiency 40–42
    following ovary removal 46–48
  role in sexual function 41, 152
  sexual dysfunction therapy 51–52, 152
    estrogen–androgen combinations 52
  see also testosterone
androstenedione 39
  changes during menopause transition 15
  changes with reproductive aging 8
anovulatory disorders 119
antidepressants, hot flash management 148–149
antihistamines, sexual dysfunction and 46

antihypertensives, sexual dysfunction and 46
apoptosis, ovarian follicle depletion and 5
L-arginine 55
aromatase inhibitors 39–40, 52
  breast cancer prevention 116
attraction, in relationships 45–46

bellergal, hot flash management 149
bicycle riding, pelvic injury and 46
bilateral oophorectomy, effects of midlife sexuality 47–48
black cohosh 153
bladder, estrogen deficiency effects 39
body fat accumulation 20–22
  HRT and 22–23
  intra-abdominal fat 21–22
  measurement of 21–22
body image 44
body mass index (BMI) 132–133
  race/ethnicity relationship 33, 133
body weight 128–129
  control 132–135
  weight gain 128
  see also obesity
bone mineral density (BMD)
  depomedroxyprogesterone (DMPA) effect 146–147
  oral contraceptive effects 147
  weight loss effect 133, 135
  see also osteoporosis
breast cancer 80–81, 109–116
  age at menopause relationship 127
  androgen association 51–52
  familial breast cancer 114–115
  nutritional factors 131–132
  prevalence 80, 109
  prevention 110–116
    aromatase inhibitors 116
    raloxifene 115–116
    tamoxifen 110–114
  risk estimation 109–110
  risk factors 81, 109, 131
    herbal therapies 153
    oral contraceptives 102
    progestins 147
  screening 80–81
Breast Cancer Prevention Trial 111–112
breast tenderness 2, 61, 66
  changes related to menopause transition 64

C-reactive protein (CRP) 21
CA-125 levels 84
calcium, dietary intake 130–131
cancer 79–80
  mortality 79
  nutritional factors 131–132
  screening 79–80
  see also specific forms of cancer
carcinoid syndrome 3
cardiovascular disease 129–130, 134
  age at menopause relationship 127
  body fat relationship 21–22
  nutritional factors 129–130
  oral contraceptive use and 101–102
  tamoxifen and 113–114
cervical cancer 81–82
  prevalence 81
  screening 81–82
chasteberry 153
childbirth injuries 46
chromosomal abnormalities
  in leiomyomas 87–88
  maternal age and 6
  reproductive aging and 9
chronic fatigue syndrome 3
cigarette smoking *see* smoking
climacteric 28
  see also menopause
clitoral changes 39
clitoral suction device 55
clomiphene citrate challenge test (CCCT) 7–8
clonidine, hot flash management 149
cognitive function 128
colorectal cancer 82–83, 131
  prevalence 82
  screening 82–83
colorectal polyps 82
communication, in relationships 45
computer assisted tomography (CT) 21–22
confounding 32–34, 59
conjugated equine estrogens (CEEs) 42, 48, 129
cortisol reaction 138
curettage 71–72
Cushing's disease 3

dehydroepiandrosterone (DHEA) 39
  sexual dysfunction therapy 54
dehydroepiandrosterone sulfate (DHEAS) 39, 54
demographics 1–2
depomedroxyprogesterone (DMPA)
  effects on bone 146–147
  hot flash therapy 146
depression 2–3, 151
  age at menopause and 1
  midlife sexuality and 46
  with premenstrual syndrome 151
diabetes 21, 130
  autonomic dysfunction 3

diagnosis 3
dietary calcium 130–131
dietary recommendations 134–136
dihydrotestosterone 39
dong quai 54, 153
drug abuse 3
dry vagina *see* vaginal dryness
dual photon X-ray absorptiometry (DXA) 21
dysfunctional uterine bleeding *see* abnormal uterine
    bleeding
dysmetabolic syndrome 134
dyspareunia 46, 49, 66

effect modification 32–34
endometrial ablation 76, 122–124
  balloon ablation 123–124
  bipolar electrosurgical ablation 123
  cryoablation 123
  laser ablation 123
  leiomyoma treatment 91
  microwave ablation 123
  rollerball ablation 123
endometrial carcinoma 69, 70, 71
  diagnosis 71
  nutritional factors 131, 132
  oral contraceptives and 100, 147
  therapy 75
endometrial hyperplasia 70, 94–95
  treatment 95
endometrial measurement 73
endometrial polyps 73–74, 94
  removal of 75
energy expenditure 19–20
estradiol
  changes during menopause transition 14, 29
  changes with reproductive aging 8, 70
  midlife sexuality and 50
  migraines and 150
  perimenopausal symptoms and 64
  race/ethnicity relationship 32–33
  see also estrogen
estrogen
  abnormal uterine bleeding and 70, 75
  changes during menopausal transition 29
  changes during reproductive aging 70
  deficiency effects on midlife sexuality 38–39, 50
    effects of ovary removal 47–48
    estrogen–androgen combination therapy 52
    sexual response 39
    urogenital atrophy 38–39
  effects on androgen bioavailability 41–42
  hot flash therapy 146
  migraine therapy 151
  see also estradiol
ethnicity
  body mass index relationship 33, 133
  hormone level relationship 32–33
exercise *see* physical activity

fatigue 3, 145
female orgasmic disorder 49
female sexual arousal disorder (FSAD) 49
fertility
    during perimenopause 148
    female age and 6
fibroids *see* leiomyomas
fibromyalgia 3
final menstrual period 2, 6, 13
fluoxetine, hot flash management 149
follicle atresia 5
    apoptosis and 5
follicle stimulating hormone (FSH) 39
    as indicator of onset of perimenopause 31
    changes during menopause transition 14, 28, 29
    changes with reproductive aging 5, 7–8, 70
    clomiphene citrate challenge test (CCCT) 7–8
    perimenopausal symptoms and 64
    race/ethnicity relationship 32–33
follistatin 28
food intake 20

Gail model for breast cancer risk estimation 109–110
genistein 132
genitourinary atrophy *see* urogenital atrophy
ginkgo biloba 55
ginseng 54, 153
gonadotropin releasing hormone (GnRH)
    pulsatility changes 7, 15, 29

headache 2, 150–151
heart disease
    body fat relationship 21
    see also cardiovascular disease
herbal therapies 152–154
    sexual dysfunction 54–55
high-density lipoprotein (HDL) 51, 129
hormone replacement therapy (HRT)
    abnormal uterine bleeding therapy 75–76
    body fat accumulation and 22–23
    effect on androgen bioavailability 41, 42, 46, 54
    hot flash therapy 146
    switching to from oral contraceptives 104
hot flashes 2, 3, 59–60, 66, 145–149
    changes related to menopause transition 64
    hormonal therapy 146–148
        dosage 148
        measuring hormone levels 148
        oral contraceptives 147–148
        progestins 146–147
    non-hormonal therapy 148–149
        alternative therapies 153
    nutritional factors 128, 154–155
    predictors of 66
    prevalence 61, 62
hypertension, oral contraceptive use and 102
hyperventilation 3
hypoactive sexual desire disorder (HSDD) 49

hypogonadotropism 3
hypothalamic–pituitary–ovarian (HPO) axis 5, 146
hysterectomy 119–121, 149
    adenomyosis treatment 94
    effects on midlife sexuality 46–48
    endometrial carcinoma treatment 75
    laparoscopic 121
    leiomyoma treatment 91–92
    long-term consequences 120
    perimenopausal symptoms and 66
hysteroscopy 72, 120, 122

ibuprofen, leiomyoma treatment 91
in vitro fertilization (IVF) 6
infertility, leiomyomas and 93
inflammation markers 21
inhibin
    changes during menopause transition 14, 28
    changes with reproductive aging 8–9
insomnia 66
    changes related to menopause transition 64
    predictors of 66
insulin resistance 130
interleukin 6 (IL-9) 21
interventional angiography 120
intra-abdominal fat 21–22
intrauterine progestin-releasing system
    abnormal uterine bleeding management 150
    leiomyoma treatment 91
isoflavones 154–155
Italian Tamoxifen Prevention Study 113

Kupperman Menopausal Index 60

laparoscopy 120, 121
    hysterectomy 121
    myolysis 121
    myomectomy 121
leiomyomas (fibroids) 74, 87–93, 119
    abnormal uterine bleeding and 69–70, 90–91
    epidemiology 88–89
    etiology 87–88
    oral contraceptives and 99
    therapy 75, 89–93
        endometrial ablation 91
        infertility 93
        intrauterine progestin-releasing system 91
        laparoscopic procedures 121
        myomectomy and hysterectomy 91–92, 121
        newly diagnosed pelvic mass 90
        pelvic pain and pressure 93
        pharmacological treatment 91
        uterine artery embolization 92–93, 121–122
levonorgestrel-releasing intrauterine system, leiomyoma
    treatment 91
libido 43–44, 152
    influencing factors 43–44
        body image 44

health/socioeconomic circumstances 43
history 44
partner availability 43
performance anxiety 44
personal well-being 43
testosterone role 40, 152
see also sexuality, in midlife
low-fat diets 129, 130, 135–136
lung cancer 84–85
prevalence 84–85
screening 85
luteinizing hormone (LH) 39, 42
changes during menopause transition 15, 28–29
changes with reproductive aging 7, 70
Lyme disease 3

magnetic resonance imaging (MRI) 21–22
mammography 80–81
masturbation 50
maternal age 6
meals, thermic effect of 19
medications, effects on midlife sexuality 46
medroxyprogesterone acetate 46, 51, 129
abnormal uterine bleeding therapy 150
breast cancer risk and 147
megestrol acetate, hot flash therapy 146
Melbourne Women's Midlife Health Project 61
men, midlife changes 42–43
menometrorrhagia 69
menopause
age at 1, 30, 127
definitions 13, 27–28
measurement validity 29–30
diagnosis 3
duration of 1, 13
hormonal changes 14–15, 42
onset 30–31
premature menopause 3
stages of 28–29
early menopause transition 2, 13
late menopause transition 2, 13
see also perimenopausal symptoms
menorrhagia 70, 91, 119
menstrual cycle
change in cycle length 6–7
irregularity 6
see also abnormal uterine bleeding
methyltestosterone 52
metrorrhagia 69
midlife 37
sexuality in *see* sexuality, in midlife
mifepristone, leiomyoma treatment 91
migraine 150–151
minimal access surgery 119–125
mutations
breast cancer 114–115
endometrial hyperplasia 95
mitochondrial DNA 9
see also chromosomal abnormalities

myocardial infarction
oral contraceptive use and 101–102
tamoxifen and 113
myomas *see* leiomyomas
myomectomy 91–92
laparoscopic 121

night sweats 2, 3, 60, 66
changes related to menopause transition 64
predictors of 66
prevalence 62
non-coital sexual pain disorder 49
norethindrone acetate 51, 55, 147
norgestimate 51
19-nortestosterone derivatives 51
nutritional factors 127–139
age at menopause and 127
cancer 131–132
cardiovascular disease 129–130
diabetes 130
dietary recommendations 134–136
osteoporosis 130–131
perimenopausal symptoms and 128
see also obesity

obesity 128–129
cancer risk and 131
diabetes and 130
oral contraceptive use and 101
weight control 132–135
see also body weight
oligomenorrhea 3, 6
oocyte donation 6
oral contraceptives (OCs) 99–104
abnormal uterine bleeding therapy 76, 99, 149, 150
beneficial effects of perimenopausal use 99–100, 147–148
breasts and 100
breast cancer risk 102
contraindications 100–102
counselling 103–104
effect on androgen bioavailability 41, 42, 46, 54
endometrial cancer risk and 100, 147
extending the active-pill period 104
hot flash therapy 146, 147–148
leiomyomas and 99
migraine management 150–151
ovarian cancer risk and 100, 147–148
side-effects 101, 103
switching to hormone replacement therapy 104
orlistat 134
osteoporosis 130–131, 134, 135
age at menopause relationship 127
see also bone mineral density (BMD)
ovarian cancer 83–84
nutritional factors 131, 132
oral contraceptives and 100, 147–148
prevalence 83
screening 84

ovarian follicles 5
  depletion of 5, 70
    apoptosis and 5
ovary removal, effects on midlife sexuality 47–48

panic disorder 3
PAP screening test 81–82
pelvic injury 46
pelvic relaxation syndrome 46
performance anxiety
  men 43
  women 44
perimenopausal symptoms 2–3, 59–66
  changes related to menopause 62–64
  measurement of 59–60
  Melbourne Women's Midlife Health Project 61
  nutritional effects 128
  predictors of 66
  risk factors 64–66
  see also specific symptoms
perimenopause 28
  onset 30–31
  see also menopause; perimenopausal symptoms
personal well-being, libido relationship 43
pheochromocytoma 3
phosphorus 131
physical activity 19, 20, 133, 136–138
  perimenopausal symptoms and 64
  stress effect on 138
phytoestrogens 129, 132
  see also soy products
polyps
  colorectal 82
  endometrial 73–74, 94
    removal of 75
post-embolization syndrome 93
postmenopause 28
power struggles 45
premature menopause 3
premature ovarian failure 5
premenstrual syndrome 151
primary adrenal failure 3
progesterone
  changes during menopause transition 14, 29
  changes with reproductive aging 8
  sexual dysfunction therapy 51
progestins
  abnormal uterine bleeding therapy 75,
    149, 150
    progestin IUDs 150
  breast cancer risk and 147
  hot flash therapy 146–147
  leiomyoma treatment 91
progestogens, sexual dysfunction therapy 51
prolactin elevation 3

race
  body mass index relationship 33, 133
  hormone level relationship 32–33

raloxifene, breast cancer prevention 115–116
  ongoing clinical trials 116
red clover 154
relationship issues see sexuality, in midlife
Remifemin 153
reproductive aging 5–10
  activin changes 9
  female age effect on fertility 6
  gonadotropin changes 7–8
  inhibin changes 8–9
  menstrual pattern changes 6–7
  ovarian follicle depletion 5, 70
  ovarian steroid changes 8
respect, lack of 45
resting metabolic rate (RMR) 19, 20
Royal Marsden Trial 112–113

St John's wort 54, 153–154
saline infusion sonohysterography 72–74, 149
selective serotonin reuptake inhibitors (SSRIs)
  effects on midlife sexuality 46
  hot flash management 149
sex hormone binding globulin (SHBG) 54
  changes during menopause transition 15
  effects on androgen bioavailability 41, 42, 54
sexual aversion disorder (SAD) 49
sexual dysfunction 42
  diagnosis of 48–50
  female orgasmic disorder 49
  female sexual arousal disorder (FSAD) 49
  herbal therapies 54–55
  non-pharmacological treatment 50
  pharmacological treatment 50–54, 55
    androgens 51–54, 152
    progestogens 51
  sexual desire disorders 49
  sexual pain disorders 49
sexuality, in midlife 38, 152
  androgen relationships 39–42
    testosterone role 40
  changes 38
  estrogen deficiency effects 38–39
    effect on sexual response 39
    urogenital atrophy 38–39
  medical issues 45–48
    hysterectomy 46–48
    medications 46
    pelvic injury 46
    surgery 46
  relationship issues 44–45
    affairs 45
    attraction 44–45
    communication 45
    power struggles/lack of respect/trust 45
  women vs men 42–43
  see also libido; sexual dysfunction
sibutramine 134
sildenafil 55
skin changes 151

sleep disturbances 3, 66, 145
   changes related to menopause transition 64
   predictors of 66
   see also night sweats
smoking 133
   age at menopause and 1, 127
   lung cancer and 84–85
   oral contraceptive use and 101, 102
socioeconomic status
   age at menopause relationship 1
   libido relationship 43
soy products 154–155
   bone loss and 131
   cancer risk and 132
   cardiovascular disease and 129
   cognitive function and 128
   diabetes and 130
   hot flashes and 128, 154–155
spontaneous abortion 6
stress 138–139
stroke, oral contraceptive use and 102
study designs 31–32
substance abuse 3, 46
surgery, midlife sexuality and 46

tamoxifen
   breast cancer prevention 110–114
      Breast Cancer Prevention Trial 111–112
      clinical use 114
      Italian Tamoxifen Prevention Study 113
      ongoing clinical trials 116
      rationale for use 110–111
      Royal Marsden Trial 112–113
   effects on healthy women 113–114
testosterone 39–40, 41
   bioavailability 41–42
   changes during menopause transition 15
   changes with age 40
   mid-cycle surge 40
   role in sexual function 40, 152

sexual dysfunction therapy 51, 52–54
   transdermal testosterone 52, 53
thermic effect of a meal 19
thyroid disease 151–152
tibolone 55
triglycerides 51, 129
trust, lack of 45
tumor necrosis factor-alpha (TNF-α) 21

ultrasonography 72–74, 149
   ovarian cancer screening 84
urogenital atrophy 2
   estrogen deficiency effects 38–39
uterine artery embolization 75, 92–93, 120, 121–122
   complications 92–93, 121–122
   contraindications 92
uterine bleeding *see* abnormal uterine bleeding

vacuum-suction curettage 71
vaginal atrophy *see* urogenital atrophy
vaginal dryness 38, 39, 50, 60, 66
   changes related to menopause transition 64
   predictors of 66
   prevalence 62
vaginismus 49
vascular reactivity 129
venlafaxine, hot flash management 148–149
venous thrombosis
   oral contraceptive use and 101
   raloxifene and 115
   tamoxifen and 113
vitamin E 154

waist-to-hip ratio 21
weight *see* body weight
well-being, libido relationship 43
wild yam cream 155

yohimbine 55, 145